M000170129

IT WILL
HAPPEN

A heart-breaking journey to
motherhood through recurrent
miscarriage and pregnancy loss

Laura Buckingham

AUSTIN MACAULEY PUBLISHERS™

LONDON • CAMBRIDGE • NEW YORK • SHARJAH

Copyright © Laura Buckingham (2020)

The right of Laura Buckingham to be identified as author of this work has been asserted by the author in accordance with section 77 and 78 of the Copyright, Designs and Patents Act 1988.

All rights reserved. No part of this publication may be reproduced, stored in a retrieval system, or transmitted in any form or by any means, electronic, mechanical, photocopying, recording, or otherwise, without the prior permission of the publishers.

Any person who commits any unauthorised act in relation to this publication may be liable to criminal prosecution and civil claims for damages.

Austin Macauley is committed to publishing works of quality and integrity. In this spirit, we are proud to offer this book to our readers; however, the story, the experiences, and the words are the author's alone.

A CIP catalogue record for this title is available from the British Library.

ISBN 9781398419650 (Paperback)
ISBN 9781398419667 (ePub e-book)

www.austinmacauley.com

First Published (2020)
Austin Macauley Publishers Ltd
25 Canada Square
Canary Wharf
London
E14 5LQ

DEDICATION

To anyone who is waiting for the rainbow after their storm.

CONTENTS

ACKNOWLEDGMENTS

Writing this personal account of our journey has been difficult at times. I started out writing down my thoughts and feelings in a blog several years ago and at the time there were only five people whom I showed it to. I guess that is where I should begin with my thank yous because without their honest feedback and support, I would never have continued writing.

I showed my husband Scoop first, after all, it is his story too and I wanted to be sure that he was happy for me to be sharing it with others. It was also a good way to open up the tough conversations between us. We've shared every part of this journey together and there were times when I thought it would break us. It didn't, it made us stronger. I feel like we could survive anything now. Scoop has his faults, as we all do. He can be grumpy at times, he snores when he is carrying a bit of extra weight and we definitely continue to have our moments but he is a wonderfully kind, interesting, patient, funny and loving husband and a superb daddy. I'm so glad he picked me (or let me pick him). I wouldn't want to be married to anyone else.

Three of my dear nursey friends, Nicola, Vikki and Katie were the next people I showed. They have all been firm supporters of mine along this journey and they remain close friends and I hope they always will. Their belief in my story-telling abilities and continued love and kindness will always be appreciated.

It was tough showing the blog to my mum as I knew that our struggles broke her heart as much they did ours. She was the fifth person I showed. I'm still not sure if she's even read all of it as I know she found parts of it too upsetting. Whether or not she read it has no actual relevance as she was with us every step of the way on this journey. I know how desperately tough she found it to sit there and watch me go through everything that I did. She felt powerless not being able to make things better for us. Thank you Ma for your ongoing love, support, Sunday lunches and homemade quilts. I don't say it enough but I love you!

Once the blog was made public, the support came flooding in from my wonderful friends and family, as well as the superb online pregnancy loss community. Thank you to this online community on Facebook and Instagram. You kept me sane when I thought I was going crazy and you helped me see the light when I was in my darkest of places.

As for the family and friends, there are too many to name personally, but a special thanks to all those who have been brave enough to have had open discussions with us about our story and those who have shared their own experiences. This is what prompted me to get going with putting 'pen to paper' and finally write the book. Getting lots of messages of support and also queries and questions made me realise that sharing all that we had been through might help others navigate their own journey.

A special thanks to 'Weird Old Aunty Lil the Lodger' who has helped me in more ways than she will ever know. Your friendship, support, love and patience has been vital to me being able to write this book.

There are a few health professionals who deserve a personal thank you. Thank you to Mr Shehata at Epsom Hospital. I wish everyone who experienced recurrent pregnancy loss could get to see you. Your knowledge and understanding around the subject is second to none. At your clinic I always felt like I was listened to and understood, and most importantly I felt that you cared. Thank you also to Dee, the nurse specialist, for all the emails, phone calls and general reassurance.

Heartfelt thanks also go to Sukhy, the kindest nurse at the EPU. You made this journey a little less awful than it could have been. If only everyone had a nurse like you looking after them. Your compassion, professionalism, knowledge and empathy make you such an asset to Darent Valley Hospital.

Thanks also to all the super stars that have helped me get my manuscript to this point. Thanks to Teresa for great suggestions and Kat for correcting my mistakes. Also to Jonesy and Lee for helping me get the manuscript ready to publish. Thank you to Katie for the cover art and illustrations, I love them. You've been as cool as a cucumber whenever we've spoken and I really hope we get to meet in person one day, for a glass of wine or two.

I owe a very big thank you to Georgia Kirke who is a bit of a pro in the field of publishing. We met through a friend over lunch one day and it was only afterwards when we were tagged in the same story on Instagram that I saw what she did for a living. I was midway through writing the book at this point but had no idea where I was going with it or how to even go about making it into something that was publishable. She has been a mentor to me during this whole process and despite a very nasty climbing injury and of course the coronavirus lockdown, she has provided ongoing support and advice. I am truly grateful for this.

Last but by no means least, I must thank my little life saver Albert Buckingham. He has been such a good sleeper and gone to bed at

6pm on the dot since he was a few months old. This has enabled me to be able to write a book while on maternity leave, something I never dreamed I would be able to do, let alone with a newborn baby.

INTRODUCTION

To think that I lived the majority of my life assuming that I actually had a choice on when I would start a family is laughable. I had absolutely no clue what I would be in for. Before embarking on my own journey to start a family I had known of a couple of people who had experienced a miscarriage or had some fertility problems. I knew that these things happened and that it wasn't always smooth running but I never really considered that I might experience these problems myself. After all, having a baby should be the most natural thing in the world. You do the deed then the egg gets fertilised. With a bit of luck on your side, in about nine months' time you become parents and are responsible for a new little life. Anyone can do it, right? You can be black or white, rich or poor (sorry, this is sounding a bit like the Only Fools and Horses theme tune). You can be educated or uneducated, in a loving relationship or playing the field. Whatever your situation, in theory you have just as good a chance as the next person of falling pregnant and growing a healthy baby. I understand that some women do not have a partner with whom they wish to take this step and other women simply do not have the desire to, but most women have the ability should they choose to do so.

I seemed to be one of those who unfortunately did not have that ability. I had a loving husband Brett, or Scoop as he is better known, but I'll come on to the reason for this later. We both had a strong desire to have children but this natural part of life did not come so naturally to us. It felt like we took knock after knock and I sometimes wonder how we kept going at times. Looking back, I can see now that we were super brave and strong although at the time I felt so fragile; mentally, physically and emotionally. Over the years my longing to have children turned to desperation. The more I struggled to have a baby, the more I wanted one. The more I saw how easy it was for others, the more I resented them but equally hated myself. I know I am not alone in feeling like this. The worlds of infertility and pregnancy loss are full of people whose arms ache for a baby. There are whole communities of people who are childless due to miscarriage and pregnancy loss and it is these people who were at the forefront of my thoughts when I wrote this book. Don't get me wrong, writing this has been incredibly therapeutic for me, if a little tough at times. It has brought up issues that I had buried and helped me process feelings that I never knew I had. Despite this I persevered because it is important for me that I share my story. My motivation for putting pen to paper has always been to help others. I feel like my job as a nurse at the hospital helped me to ask the right questions, speak to the appropriate people and, rightly or wrongly so, I think it gave me a bit of a head start when it came to getting answers. It is probably thanks to this that I have my happy ending and by sharing my experiences I hope that I can help others to get theirs too. I want to at least try to make the journey there a little bit less lonely. I would love nothing more than this book to provide people with some answers, reasons, suggestions, but more importantly companionship and hope. I have written the book that I think would have helped me during the times when I didn't know where to turn.

People would tell me all the time that 'it will happen'. But how did they know that? Could they be certain? There was a time when these well-meant words from others gave me hope and encouragement but after hearing them so many times, I stopped believing them. This phrase no longer brought hope for me but having come out of the other side of that horrendous journey, I can see now that they were right. It did happen for me but I am all too aware that this is not the case for everyone. My story could have had such a different ending. There were some pivotal moments when I felt like giving up on my hopes of having a baby but somehow I found the determination to persevere, be it due to my stubbornness, desperation, ambivalence or sheer foolhardiness.

I am thrilled to say that I am now mum to a rainbow baby and am currently navigating motherhood after miscarriage, which comes with its own set of challenges. But before that, you probably want to hear more about the journey we went on to get to this point. It was 2012 when we started trying for a baby. This is the story of our struggle to start a family...

ABOUT YOU

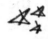

Throughout the book I have included some activities and questions in an 'ABOUT YOU' section for your consideration. My hope is that because I found writing so helpful that you may also benefit. It is completely up to you if you write or simply reflect and it can be for your eyes only or shared with others. This is your book. You do what suits you. Not all of it will be relevant to all readers but I hope it helps you make sense of your journey and it supports you to process your feelings.

Firstly, before we get started with my story you might want to have a think about what you would say to yourself if you could go back in time to before your baby making journey began. What would you write in a letter to your younger self about your journey so far?

_____

_____

_____

_____

_____

_____

_____

THE DOUBLE-EDGED SWORD OF

BEING OPEN

Scoop and I had been together for a little over four years on 24th October 2012 when I went to the doctor to have my contraceptive implant removed so we could begin trying for a baby. We had often spoken about having a family and due to wanting four children we thought we'd better get started sooner rather than later so that we would have babies around the same time as our friends. Well, I did anyway, and I had managed to persuade Scoop. After all, I was 27 and my biological clock was ticking. We weren't married as we couldn't afford the wedding that we wanted so thought we would wait and have a wedding at a later date. I was happy to have a little registry office ceremony followed by a party down the local rugby club but Scoop wanted a big 'do' with all our family and friends and wouldn't entertain any other ideas. So the idea of a big wedding was put on hold and having a family was our current priority. We (mainly I) were very excited about it.

We hadn't really discussed having a baby with anyone else prior to me having the implant removed. Why would we? - you might wonder. After all it was our business, not anyone else's. However, I am a very open person and can't help but discuss all the details of my life with those close to me and sometimes even with those who are not so close. I've always been that way. Pretty handy really, considering that right now I am writing about the most sad and vulnerable times of our lives and will be publishing it for all and sundry to read. Little did I know that my openness would stand us in good stead throughout the next few years of our life. How can people support you when they don't know what you are going through? Having said that, as you can imagine it wasn't always beneficial having everyone know exactly what we were going through. It was probably my feelings of excitement that meant that I couldn't help but tell the world and his wife that we were now trying for a baby. I was old enough, in a secure job having qualified as a nurse earlier in the year and we were in a loving relationship. Having a baby naturally seemed like the next step in our grand life plans. By the time my mum was 27 she already had a seven- and five-year-old and was pregnant with a third baby. I had always imagined starting a family in my mid-to-late twenties so in my opinion we were right on schedule.

I am the eldest of three children. I have a brother who is two years younger and a sister who is eight years younger. I am lucky enough to have a large extended family with lots of aunties, uncles and cousins. Growing up was so much fun in my family. There were big gatherings on special occasions and regular get-togethers too. They oozed fun, love and laughter. I looked forward to good times recreating old traditions and starting new ones with my children and their cousins. It's funny how you imagine your life and envisage the future. I had thought a lot about having a baby and I pictured our life together as a family. Since the age of 14 I had dreamt about having babies and always believed that it was my real purpose in life. I never really thought about a career, I just wanted to be a mum. I had a list of baby names in my Year 9 homework diary and dreamt about marrying someone who would be a fantastic dad and having a big, happy family that lived on a farm. I was going to have two boys and two girls, named Bertie, Ted, Connie and Flo and they would be born in that order. I think this longing for a large family developed from my love of watching Little House on the Prairie!

I had never considered us having difficulties with the getting pregnant part and didn't ever think about the fact that I might not actually be able to have a family. My mum had always told me how all the women in the family were incredibly fertile so it never occurred to me that I would be any different. As the eldest, I always imagined that I would be the first of my siblings to have a baby. We were super excited and in hindsight probably incredibly cocky about the prospect of becoming parents. After my contraceptive implant removal, it was only a couple of months until Christmas 2012 arrived. We imagined having a baby in the family next year and thought about how special it would be and how we would get to dress the baby up in cute little outfits and sign their name on the Christmas cards. We spoke openly to our families about this and we were all excited about the year ahead.

When the doctor was removing my implant that day, I asked him when the effect of it would wear off and was told that when I woke up the next morning that it would be as if the implant was never there. So this was it then. It was time to start baby making. It was a strange feeling having spent my earlier years trying not to get pregnant. A real fear and anxiety was instilled in me when I was a teenager and yet here I was actually trying to have a baby. Naively we assumed it would happen for us in no time at all. Now, everyone knows that babies are made when two people who love each other…only kidding! There is no need to go into the details here. We all know how babies are made. Or do we? I'm sure that most people lay back and think of England and within a few months they get their big fat positive (BFP). *I have no idea why a positive pregnancy test is referred to as a BFP in the TTC (trying to conceive) community, but it is. In fact there are many acronyms that are used. A summary of the most common ones can be found at the end of the book.* Tommy's, the baby charity, said in 2018 that about one in three women will conceive within a month of starting to try and more than 8 out of 10 couples where the woman is aged under 40 will be pregnant within a year (Tommy's, 2018). This is assuming they are having regular unprotected sex. It wasn't that easy for us to conceive. Before we were even off the starting blocks we appeared to be on the wrong side of the statistics. We were in the less than 20% that did not fall pregnant within a year of trying to conceive.

After a few months of TTC with no success, it appeared to be normal practice to download various Apps, start tracking menstrual cycles and doing ovulation tests. This is what I did. It became a bit of an obsession. Sex is scheduled, body temperatures are monitored and cervical mucus is analysed. If you are new to all this then it may be too much information but this is only just scratching the surface of what women go through to make sure they BD (bed down / baby dance / do the deed / shag) at the most optimal time. Romance is pretty limited when operation baby making is in full swing. I had an app on my phone that showed a tree branch on the homepage and on the fertile days some pink flowers would appear on the branch. When the flowers appeared I would drop hints all evening. I tried to be subtle because I was conscious of making our sex life too regimented. Over time I would come to learn that I just had to say, "flowers are on the branch" to make it clear what needed to happen. What a turn on that must have been! The TWW (two week wait) is the time between ovulation and the arrival of a period. It is a bloody awful time when TTC. You BD on the right days and just have to wait to see if you were successful. Every little symptom makes you think this might be your month, it's a bit like torture. Pre-menstrual symptoms are incredibly similar to early pregnancy symptoms. Sore boobs, cramps, discharge, nausea and hot flushes are symptoms that can leave you hoping, wondering and second guessing until the menstrual period begins. Even after getting a BFN (Big Fat Negative) there is still a bit of hope that you could just be testing too early and its only when Aunt Flo (AF- period) finally rears her ugly red head that it is confirmed that you are 'out' that month. When this occurs month after month you really can begin to detest old Aunty Flo!

My 2013 flew by, just like any other year. There was nothing particularly terrible and nothing overly exciting. It consisted of shift work, home renovations, and nights out with friends, weddings, hen weekends, a summer holiday to France and lots of dog walks. Our dog Cooper is our little fur baby and I truly don't know how I, and more so Scoop, would have coped over the years without the unconditional love from our little ginger prince #cooperthegingerstaffy. 2013 also involved a lot of that monitoring, tracking and scheduling when it came to the baby making stuff. In fact, it was this that resulted in me ending up knowing my body so well that I could tell when I was ovulating without even using the tests and, believe it or not, it was even possible to tell which ovary I had ovulated from. It did indeed become an obsession, which caused a lot of friction between us and put a strain on our relationship. Infertility is full of feelings of guilt and shame. We didn't know why we weren't falling pregnant. Was it Scoop's fault or my fault? We both felt inadequate, like we were failing the other and letting each other down. Or were we just incompatible? You do hear of things like that happening; opposite blood types or something similar. I think Scoop would have preferred it if we had kept our TTC plans to ourselves. We (mainly I) had put a lot of pressure on ourselves by telling everyone that we were trying for a baby. We would constantly get asked if I was expecting yet and people would try to second guess if we had good news to share. I think most people were just excited for us as opposed to simply being nosey, but it did get annoying. As I mentioned, I had not considered having difficulties TTC so it never crossed my mind that we would spend months and years answering questions about our fertility and justifying why we didn't have a baby yet. It was at these times that I regretted being so open; however, when the knocks started coming our way I couldn't have been gladder that people knew what we were going through. There were times when the support was vital. There was another good thing to come from our openness. Not only did we receive support from others when it was so desperately needed, but we were also able to provide support for others going through similar situations. It wasn't even any specific support that we provided but by being open about our own experiences, it opened up the dialogue and made the difficult conversations a little easier with and for others. It helped make people feel less alone in their struggles and it created friendships and communities that would otherwise not have been formed. In hindsight, the openness probably contributed towards our stress levels but weighing it all up, I would do the same again. I would maybe try to keep the TTC part under wraps a little better but regarding the pregnancies and losses I wouldn't change a thing.

Thanks to everyone around us knowing what we were going through, there was also a lot of well-meant advice received. Everyone knows someone who struggled to conceive and everyone wants to share what worked for them. We were offered many pearls of wisdom. Some people would suggest having sex every day, others would say every other day, but our GP

19

recommended every third day. We were advised to stop trying so hard and stop thinking about it; people said I was getting too stressed. Some people suggest acupuncture and other (what I like to call) 'airy fairy shit', but the 'best' advice came from an older family member. She told me that when she finally conceived her son it had been thanks to putting her bum up the headboard and legs in the air in order to give the little swimmers the assistance of gravity. She suggested that I use the same technique. It was a pretty cringey moment when she told me this while we were sat in the garden with the whole family one Sunday afternoon, digging into BBQ food. We did think it was hilarious but I would be lying if I said we didn't give it a go! I'd have given anything a shot.

I started noticing that I was jealous of other women who seemed to be getting pregnant easily, or in some cases by mistake. I questioned why it was happening for them and not for us. *When would it be our turn?* My frustration levels built and my confidence took a nose dive. I felt insecure and ashamed of my inability to do what other women could so easily do. I thought about the women whose bodies are under extreme pressure, those considered unhealthy, those living in terrible circumstances and how they can still get pregnant. I couldn't help but wonder if there was something wrong with me.

I had sought some advice about what to do if you couldn't get pregnant and was told that after a year of TTC with no luck, the GP would do some basic tests and investigations. As the festive season approached I admitted defeat and booked an appointment to start this process in the new year. I was so scared that they were going to find something wrong with me, but equally hopeful that if there was that it would be a quick fix.

ABOUT YOU

How did you imagine your family set up? At what age did you plan to start trying for a baby? What age gaps would you have preferred between your children? Did you have any ideas about preferred gender or names? Or was that just me?

_____

_____

_____

_____

_____

If it has not worked out how you had imagined, how does that make you feel? _____

_____

_____

_____

_____

_____

GETTING OFF THE STARTING BLOCKS

I believe Christmas Eve fell on a Tuesday in 2012. It was three days after my work Christmas party. Oh the work Christmas party. If I remember rightly, I don't actually remember much of the night. It was a long time ago now but if I am completely honest, my reason for the lack of memory is because I was shit faced! I'll tell you what I do remember. Just before leaving the house, dressed as a Christmas elf nonetheless (elf shoes too), I popped to the loo and lo and behold AF had arrived. Fucking fabulous! I hated periods more now than ever before. It's not just the whole bleeding and cramping for five poxy days and the bad skin, bloating and chocolate cravings. No, it's a reminder. AF now also meant that we didn't get pregnant AGAIN that month! It was bloody typical that it would come early too and on the night of the party as well. Great! It was only a tiny smear on the tissue but I

22

knew that I didn't have long until the red river was in full flow. Unfortunately, in my fluster to get out of the door on time I forgot to grab extra supplies for the night. Fortunately, when I arrived at my friend's house she gave me some tampons which I shoved in the pocket of my handbag and we headed to the party together.

The Christmas party involved a crappy buffet, lots of drinking, over the top dancing and plenty of shop talk. Then I did what everyone wishes they didn't do at a work party, I got emotional. I was upset about the whole (no) pregnancy thing and after over a year of trying, tracking and testing, things were clearly getting to me. My work mates knew what I was going through and being in the rather squiffy state that I was, I ended the night lying on the floor outside the hotel on one of my colleagues laps, sobbing, while waiting for my taxi. There was even a rendition of Whitney Houston's Greatest Love of All. 'I believe that children are our future' and all that. There I was, on the 21st December, blubbing to my work friends at our Christmas party, about my infertility! What a dick!

Anyhow, fast forward a few days to Christmas Eve and I was still suffering from the after effects of the party. I'm not great with hangovers. I called my friend who was coming to visit us later in the day with my goddaughter. We had planned to watch the Santa parade around our estate, as per tradition, but I wanted to give them the heads up that I was sick. Although I was pretty sure it was a hangover and not a bug, I thought they should stay away just in case because I didn't want them to get sick and ruin their Christmas.

After chatting on the phone to my friend, she had another idea about what could be wrong with me. Although this was the month that we had tried the infamous legs in the air technique, I knew I couldn't be pregnant because I had my period already. Didn't I?

Well actually it had stopped that night of the Christmas party and was yet to return again. Thinking about it, I had not had to use any of those supplies from the pocket in my handbag, it had just been that one smear before going out that night. Scoop was sent to the shops to buy a pregnancy test. I didn't actually believe that I could be pregnant, it was more about ruling it out.

I went in to the toilet, followed the instructions and when I saw the test I called Scoop upstairs to look at it too. We could not believe our eyes when we saw a plus sign. It was bloody positive. We cried and hugged. A lot. This was the best Christmas present we could have ever wished for. We had waited all this time but finally we did it! We later found out that the bleeding that I had mistaken for my period was actually called implantation bleeding which is very commonly mistaken for an early light period. We told my friend about the pregnancy when she came over with my goddaughter for the Santa parade but other than that we kept the news to ourselves.

We went out that night for drinks with friends and I was bursting to tell everyone but we had decided to wait until 12 weeks because that's what people did. This seems to have become the social norm back in the 1970s when the ultrasound and screening tests became commonplace at around the 11–14 week mark. Prior to these medical developments women would become aware of their pregnancy after a missed period or two but would hold back from announcing until they could feel foetal movements at around four months. I could not wait that long and by all accounts pregnancy was going to be tough. What with all the morning sickness and fatigue, I wondered if I would need the support of my friends, family and colleagues before 12 weeks. We discussed it but agreed that everyone already knew that we were trying for a baby so it would be nice to keep this as our little secret, even if I was bursting to tell everyone that I was finally up the duff!

On Christmas day I woke up without a hangover (for the first time in a good few years, I was like a changed woman) and we went to Scoop's best mate's house for breakfast as per tradition. We hadn't even walked over the threshold when they announced that they were expecting their second baby. It was early days and they had only just found out. Well, do you think we could keep our own news to ourselves? Hell no! We shared our news too and it was a very excitable Christmas morning. We were due in August only days apart from each other. What a way to start Christmas day. I had been dreading it but actually it was panning out pretty well so far. We could not wipe the smiles off our faces.

We were at my mum's for dinner on Christmas Day and as usual there was a full house. I have a brother and a sister and a step brother and sister. At the time we were all adults with partners but no children, so Christmas was usually about having a good old knees up. When we arrived the champagne was flowing. I was offered a glass, which I took and just held. I swapped my drink with Scoop's a couple of times and pretended to drink from the glass which never emptied. Soon we realised that there was no way we would be able to keep it a secret from this lot all day. My mum pretty much guessed after I declined some pâté. She screamed with excitement so everyone who was there knew what was happening and within the hour she had phoned her mum and brothers to inform the whole extended family. So much for keeping it quiet until after the 12-week scan. We felt bad that my dad and my in-laws were not aware so we told them too. We sent them pictures of us holding the positive test. Everyone was so excited for us. It was the best Christmas ever! We talked about our baby all day long. We couldn't wait to see who the baby would look like and to decide on a name. We already had so many hopes and dreams for the future. Anyone who has had a positive pregnancy test can understand these feelings. We dreamt about the person that they would become and how our lives would change. It was all we could think and talk about.

I had the usual early pregnancy symptoms of sore boobs, extreme fatigue and waves of nausea. I desperately wanted to have actual morning sickness as opposed to just feeling sick, simply for reassurance purposes. Apparently this nausea is completely normal and only a very low percentage of women have actual sickness. So instead I spent a lot of time going to and from the bathroom thinking I was going to be sick but never was. I ended up telling my work colleagues our news. Working as a nurse on the wards meant that in order to protect myself and the baby from coming to any harm, I had to inform the people that I worked with so that I didn't have to care for high-risk patients. They were all very excited for me as well as being supportive and understanding when I would spend the first hour or two of every shift in and out of the loo and dry heaving.

Life had suddenly got sweeter and everything became more colourful now that we were expecting a baby. I would think about it all day and dream about it all night. My mind was fully occupied by this little thing growing inside me and I couldn't be happier. I had self-referred to the hospital for my maternity care. I soon received my midwife appointment for when I would be eight weeks and we awaited the appointment letter for the all-important dating scan. I was so excited to see our little bubba that I started researching private scan clinics so I could get a sneaky peak.

13 days after the BFP was the 6th January. I was nine hours into working the 12.5-hour day shift when my world came crashing down. I went to the loo. There was blood on the tissue paper. When I saw it my heart sank and all I could manage to do was say 'oh shit' out loud to myself before breaking down in tears. When I appeared from the toilet my colleagues were amazing. They

tried to reassure me that spotting can be normal in early pregnancy. They phoned the EPU (early pregnancy unit) but they wouldn't see me unless a referral was made. Our Matron walked with me down to A&E where they tested my urine and referred me to EPU. Whilst sat waiting in A&E I tried to stop myself from sobbing because I felt like a fool for being so dramatic. It was a familiar place to me but on this day it seemed like somewhere new and scary. I was still wearing my uniform so everyone who walked past, staff and patients alike, took a second glance. Those who knew me came to see if I was okay but that only made me cry more. A scan was arranged for me at the EPU for the following morning so I was sent home and reassured that spotting can be completely normal. I phoned Scoop to let him know what was happening and he remained positive. I couldn't. Of course I hoped with all my heart that everything would be okay but I didn't believe that it would be. We didn't share this with anyone outside of a few people at my work who needed to know. We thought it best to wait and see what the scan showed the next day and didn't want to upset anyone unnecessarily. I have no memory of what we did at home that night. None at all.

The next day we arrived at the EPU for the scan. I still felt very pregnant, maybe everything would be okay. I was new to this so did not know what to expect. Due to being only seven weeks pregnant (based on my LMP, last menstrual period), I required a trans-vaginal (TV) ultrasound scan. This involves a probe that resembles a light saber being inserted into the foofie. They dim the lights and the room is barely lit by the monitor screen. A giant condom type thing and a shed load of lube are put on the wand before it is inserted. Then you watch the screen, waiting to see the flicker of a heartbeat. We watched the screen and we waited. And waited.

I have never felt as vulnerable as I did in that moment. That was the moment that I changed forever. That moment they said 'I'm sorry, there is no heartbeat'. My heart was broken.

The appointment letter for our dating scan arrived a few days later. I just sobbed.

ABOUT YOU

Do you think that this journey has changed you? If so, how have you changed? Do you wish you could go back to being the person you were before?

_____

_____

_____

_____

_____

_____

_____

_____

_____

_____

_____

_____

SELF-LOATHING

Our 2014 didn't get off to the best start. Following the miscarriage in January we got straight back to it and fortunately fell pregnant again on the next cycle. Once again we used the legs in the air method. Although I later found out that apparently this makes no difference because the silly sperm swim around in different directions anyway. It is, in fact, the female body that does most of the work. The uterus muscles contract to coax the sperm to where it needs to be. This sounds to me a lot like marriage and actually life in general; the man being guided by the woman. We had been told that you are extremely fertile after a miscarriage so made the most of this opportunity. Everyone reassured me that having a miscarriage is very common and that everything would be okay next time. But unfortunately the same thing happened and we miscarried again, this time on Valentine's Day.

I couldn't help but blame myself. I blamed the first miscarriage on my drunken state at the work Christmas party and I was sure that the one in February was caused by the heavy bass at a Rudimental gig we went to at Brixton Academy the night before the bleeding began. We asked the doctor if this was the cause and they said that it was very unlikely. When I asked them what they thought the cause was they couldn't actually tell me. They said that it was probably just bad luck, but I couldn't help but doubt myself. I thought that it might be because I was stressed at work and had been working long hours or maybe because I went for a run too soon after the last miscarriage. I even considered the fact that we weren't married or that we had initially been so cocky about having a baby might be the reason we had miscarried. In fact, most causes of miscarriage are either unknown or out of our control and very rarely does anything that you do or don't do affect this. Whatever the reason was, I couldn't accept bad luck as the answer. I wanted a proper scientific reason, something I could work with, something we could fix, and until we got that I would blame myself. I found myself guilty until proven innocent.

How could I have been so silly to get my hopes up this time? I felt terribly guilty. I was so worried that Scoop blamed me too, so much so that I couldn't bring myself to discuss it with him because I wouldn't have coped with having those fears confirmed. The consultant told us that many people have one miscarriage and to have two was actually quite common too. Once again I was reassured that it was likely that all would be well next time, this time the reassurance came from a health professional so I held on to this. Third time lucky and all that! My GP wouldn't run the tests that we had talked about a few months before because it was now clear that I had no problem getting pregnant. I tried to see this as a positive; maybe it was just a numbers game. I could get pregnant; it was just a matter of having one that stuck. We now had to conceive again and cross our fingers that it would work out and stay put this time.

Over the course of the year we went to a lot of weddings, ten to be precise. We have been to a lot of weddings as a couple but this would be our busiest year, with four in the 6-week school summer holidays. It was lots of fun but due to finances and limited annual leave, we were unable to go on holiday, other than a long weekend to Ireland which happened to be for another wedding. Now I do love a wedding, but this year I found myself dreading them. Well, I didn't dread the wedding itself, it was the announcement of the pregnancy which usually followed three to six months later. I'd sit there watching two of our friends or family saying their vows and almost resenting them a little because I just knew that they would get pregnant and have a baby before us. Thinking back now it was an incredibly paranoid assumption. I would anticipate it happening and then during the six months or so after the wedding I would avoid seeing or talking to people just in case they told me they were pregnant. This was a real anxiety and fear for me. My jealousy was becoming an issue. To begin with I was able to fake some enthusiasm and tended to react with a very over the top 'congratulations' but people soon saw through this, or at least I thought they did. When someone announced their pregnancy to me I would make my excuses and then usually spend the rest of the day in a mood and end up sobbing in the shower or into my pillow that night. I remember going through a stage of hearing people announce their pregnancies while in the same room, like at work on the ward or at a party for example, and I couldn't acknowledge it at all. I would completely ignore the fact that I had overheard their news because that prevented me from having to react to it and fake my happiness for them. I asked my friends and family to just tell me by text, that way I had a little time to process my thoughts, be angry, sad or jealous and then speak to them when I had gotten over the initial shock and had my game face on. It wasn't that I was angry, sad or jealous because of them or their baby. I was angry, sad and jealous that it worked for them and not us. It just broke my heart.

As our first due date arrived I began to struggle more. Scoop's best mate and his partner had their second little boy in August. We should have been having ours too. It felt so unfair. However, my jealousy and bitterness dissipated once the baby had arrived. He was so wonderful and we were happy for them, just terribly sad for ourselves.

Things got increasingly difficult, mentally and emotionally, after our third pregnancy loss. It was the 3rd September when we got out BFP. 'Third time lucky' we thought. We kept the news to ourselves this time because the disappointment and sadness was taking its toll on our family and friends too. We wanted to be able to give them good news. We had managed to get a reassurance scan at the EPU for six weeks. Once again I had the sore boobs and early pregnancy fatigue but no morning sickness. Although I knew this didn't usually start for another couple of weeks yet, it still made me anxious and I presumed the worst. When we went in for the scan we were seen by the same nurse that had scanned me the last two times and she had been the one to tell us that there was no heartbeat previously. I guess this would normally be quite triggering for some people; however, I knew this nurse quite well as she had been my mentor when I was a student nurse on the gynaecology ward. I respect her and trust her implicitly. Knowing our history she was anxious for us too but she remained calm and professional. I will be forever thankful to her for all the support and care she has shown us over the years.

Once again I was too early on in the pregnancy to have a tummy scan so I had to make sure I had an empty bladder for the TV scan. There I lay, legs akimbo and light saber inserted. Scoop and I held

33

hands and looked at each other while she began scanning me. Within a few seconds she was able to confirm that there was a pregnancy in the uterus and she could see a heartbeat. I honestly did not believe her because I couldn't hear anything. I looked at the screen and I could see a little blob and inside the blob was a little flicker. A flickering, beating heart! Apparently it was too early to hear it but it could be seen. It was absolutely amazing. I can still picture it now. Everything looked as it should and the measurements were correct. This really was our 'third time lucky'. The nurse hugged us and booked us in for the next scan in a couple of weeks. We went straight to my mum's house to tell her the good news. We were planning to keep it a secret for a little longer but we were so excited that we had to share our news with someone. When we told my mum that we were pregnant again she seemed excited but equally nervous. She seemed to be holding back a little, that was until we told her that we had already had a scan and seen a heartbeat. Then her reaction changed. She was excited and I could tell she was over the moon for us, for all of us. It was the good news that we had all been waiting for. I had done my research and apparently if you get to the point of a heartbeat there is a significantly lowered chance of miscarriage. Things were looking positive. Despite this, it was a very nerve-wracking time. I constantly doubted my symptoms, or lack thereof. At the 8-week scan the measurements were correct and the heartbeat was strong. For the first time we heard our baby's heart beating. We had now passed the point of the previous losses. It was all starting to feel real and we couldn't believe that it was finally happening for us. I had my dating scan already booked for 14 weeks and the early pregnancy unit offered me one last reassurance scan before then. Of course I accepted. I wanted to see this precious bubba as many times as I possibly could. Scoop said that my mum could go with me instead of him as he had already seen the baby twice and would be seeing it again at the dating scan; plus, he was struggling to keep getting the time off work. My mum was so excited.

At 11 weeks, it would be the first time I would have a tummy scan instead of the trans-vaginal scan, like the many others that came before it. I had to have a full bladder for this type of scan so sat in the waiting room with my mum, downing water and actually looking forward to the scan for the first time. I was excited to show off my baby's beating heart to its grandma and my mum was super excited to meet her first grandchild. My belly was getting bigger and I was showing already so couldn't wait to finally admit to being pregnant and fat as opposed to just fat. I remember sitting in the waiting room for the EPU and couldn't help but wonder about the other women in there. I had sat there several times before and gone into the room to receive bad news. I felt bad for being in the same waiting room, I felt guilty that these poor women had to share a waiting room with me because I was happy and had a baby growing inside me and they might be getting bad news like I had before. I always thought that they should have separate waiting rooms so that women who are going through losses shouldn't have to sit and watch happy women stroking their bellies. Yet here I was on the other side of it, but I didn't stroke my belly. I knew what it felt like to witness it.

When we went in, the nurse began to scan my tummy but she wasn't able to get a good picture. Like I said before, I had never had a tummy scan myself but I had heard others being asked to empty their bladder before. After a few minutes of attempting to scan me, she asked me to pop to the loo and have a wee so they could do an internal trans-vaginal scan. She wasn't getting a very good picture, probably because I had drunk too much water and my bladder was *too* full. I jumped down from the couch and left the room to go to the toilet. I shouldn't have been too concerned given that I was aware that this was normal practice, but I was. I didn't (couldn't) look at my mum as I left the room and I acted as

35

if everything was tickety-boo. However, as I was sat on the toilet having a wee I knew what was about to happen. I had an overwhelming feeling of sadness – I knew it had all been too good to be true. You know that gut feeling you get? That feeling of doom? Like the floor has been wiped from beneath you. I just knew what they were about to tell me and I could not shake that feeling. It took everything I had not to cry. I knew if I started I wouldn't be able to stop. I considered doing a runner so I could be ignorant to the truth. I wanted to escape the EPU and the hospital for that matter so I could just pretend that everything was still okay. I didn't want to come out of the toilet and I certainly did not want to go back into that room to face my mum and the nurse and that bloody light saber, but I did. I put on my game face and smiled at my mum and the nurse as I re-entered the room and noticed there was now another nurse and a doctor in the room too. It was almost as if everything was happening in slow motion. I hoped and prayed that my gut feeling was wrong and that all this fuss was just because I had drunk too much water and my bladder was obscuring the view. I hoped and prayed that we were about to see the heartbeat and my mum and my baby would make each other's acquaintance. I couldn't go through another loss, not this time. I wasn't sure I could cope with it.

I felt so vulnerable lying there. As I undressed and got back on the couch the nurse looked at me with a concerned face and asked me if I understood what was happening to which I responded with a smile and nod while the tears filled up in my eyes and a lump began forming in my throat. The nurse took her time to look around properly and made sure she was certain of the result before she gave it to me. I lay silently weeping with tears streaming down my face while the nurse told me how sorry she was that the heartbeat could not be detected. I could hear my mum sobbing the other side of the curtain. I couldn't believe that this was happening to me again. I felt like I was being punished for being hopeful and optimistic. It turned out that my baby's heart had stopped beating the day after the eight-week scan, which meant I had a dead baby inside me for three weeks and I didn't know. How did I not know? I would learn that this is what is called a missed miscarriage (MMC). My body still thought it was pregnant. I hated my body. Why couldn't it do what it was meant to do? I hated myself. I must have done something wrong. I have never felt like such a failure.

My mum's sobbing turned to wailing and I remember just trying to focus on her. I told her to calm down and to stop being so embarrassing. I can't believe I said that to her, I feel so bad. I don't think I was in denial about what was happening, I just didn't want to process this news just yet and my mum's heartbreak distracted me from my own, for a little while at least. We were ushered from the scanning room past the waiting room to somewhere with more privacy. I was one of those poor women that you would observe from the waiting room, once again receiving bad news. The nurse kept asking me if I understood what was happening, to which I would just nod. What followed was a bit of a blur. I phoned Scoop to tell him what had happened and he left work and came straight to the hospital.

I was booked in the next day for an operation to have the 'products' removed. This was called an evacuation of retained products of conception (ERPC). This terminology is horrible. The name has since changed and it is now called a Surgical Management of Miscarriage (SMM). Although, I have to say that the word miscarriage itself is not much better. It suggests that the blame lies with the mother, as if she was almost careless and didn't carry her precious cargo properly. Of course this is very rarely the case.

I had to have the operation because my body was not letting go of the pregnancy itself so it would need to be surgically removed and sent off for testing. There are other management options; however, I would come to learn at a later date why the surgical management option was advised in my case. I'd never had an operation before, and I was terrified that I wouldn't wake up or that I'd be able to feel it. Of course both of these things were very unlikely to happen but I was in a high state of anxiety and despair so my thoughts were by no means rational. That night before the operation we went home and we sobbed. We really thought this time it was going to work but it wasn't to be and we were devastated. Having seen the heartbeat twice and reaching 11 weeks, we were rather confident. We had been telling more and more people and even dared to let ourselves have a wander around Mothercare talking about prams, cots and the like. I even bought a pair of little new-born teddy bear booties; how could I have been so silly? Most people would see this as a natural thing to do when coming up to 12 weeks, but I should have held off and waited until we were sure that everything was okay. I felt like an idiot. I should have seen this coming.

We had a lot of phone calls to make to inform people what had happened but I couldn't face telling anyone, not in person anyway. I sent a few texts to friends but left Scoop to tell everyone else. Bless him, he must have found that so difficult. I was sure he resented me for putting him through all this again. All I could say was, 'I'm sorry'. I felt bad for my mum too. She would have to call around her friends and the wider family to tell them. I wondered if she was ashamed of me and my inability to carry a baby, to provide her with a grandchild. I was letting her down. I felt like I was letting everyone down.

My body had failed me once again. It highlighted my failings as a woman and caused me to feel incredibly embarrassed and ashamed. *What kind of woman can't have a baby?* I resigned myself to the fact that my body obviously didn't work properly and I was basically a shit female. I wondered what people thought of me and hoped that they didn't feel sorry for me, I couldn't bear that. When we told them our sad news we received so much love back from all the people who cared about us. I guess this is why telling people about the pregnancy in the first place is so important to me. It means that there is a network of support there for you if and when (in our case just *when*) things do go wrong. It is important that you have that support, for both of you. I didn't want sympathy or pity though. All I really wanted was a baby and no one could make that happen for us, but just knowing that people were there and cared about us was enough.

The whole experience was very traumatic and we started wondering if we would ever have a baby. We got up early the following morning after very little sleep and went to the hospital where I was prepped for theatre. I had sore boobs, nausea and heartburn. I still felt pregnant, it was so cruel. Maybe I was still pregnant, I wondered. Maybe they had got it wrong. I remember thinking that surely they should scan me again to check, just in case. My mind was all over the place, it wasn't fair, it felt so unjust.

I was wearing nothing but a gown and stockings as I was pushed through the corridors of the hospital by a familiar-faced porter. This hospital was also my place of work and I felt like everyone knew my business, I just wanted to be anonymous for once. I was operated on in the morning of 22nd October 2014. When I came round from the anaesthetic I was incredibly emotional, which is quite common anyway, let alone in these circumstances. I was discharged later that day and took a couple of weeks off work after this which I really needed for both my physical and mental recovery. Our world seemed so grey again. Deep down I knew that to lose three babies within a year wasn't just bad luck. I hoped that we could begin to investigate why this was happening and do something to stop it from happening again. We waited to hear about an appointment to discuss moving forward with testing. Life went on, people around me continued to get pregnant and everyone prepared for the Christmas festivities.

Six weeks later, on 18th December 2014, I had a phone call from the early pregnancy unit while I was at work. They had phoned upstairs to the unit that I worked on to inform me that the results of the testing they had done on the 'products' of the last miscarriage were back. They requested my presence in the EPU right away. I knew this couldn't be good news but had no idea about what was to come. I made my apologies to my boss and hurried down there. I called Scoop quickly on my way to the unit and promised to call him back as soon as I knew anything. I was greeted by my favourite nurse who gave me an awkward smile and ushered me into the room where the consultant sat at the desk with a pile of leaflets. When I awkwardly joked with him that things looked a bit serious I was told that they were and he gestured for me to take a seat.

It turned out that the tests showed that I had what was called a molar pregnancy. Now there are two types of molar pregnancies: complete and partial. I had a partial molar pregnancy (PMP). This is where an egg is fertilised by two sperm resulting in an embryo that is incompatible with life due to it having 69 chromosomes instead of 46. So, my baby was never going to grow into a baby. That baby that I dreamt about and made all those plans for would not have developed properly and would never have survived. I wasn't sure if this made it easier to deal with or not. I was just so shocked initially but thinking back to the day of the scan when I was with my mum, I remembered that the nurse had mentioned this, hence why the surgical management was advised. In fact, the nurse had even given me a leaflet about it but I must have misplaced it with all the other paperwork. I think I remembered flicking through it and reading something about cancer and chemotherapy and dismissed it, assuming she had given it to me error. I had just found out I was miscarrying. That whole day was a blur.

They explained that the nurse had initially thought that it was a molar pregnancy on the day of the scan, due to the appearance of the placenta. It appears like a bunch of grapes on the ultrasound scan and the cells continue to grow rapidly and keep growing even after the heartbeat has stopped. This would have been why my tummy was getting bigger despite the baby not growing and therefore why I was showing so early on in the pregnancy. The cells tend to embed deeply into the lining of the womb and can sometimes spread to other organs of the body, turning cancerous and requiring chemotherapy or even a hysterectomy in extreme cases. Due to these risks, I required follow up blood and urine tests by the haemato-oncology unit at Charing Cross Hospital in London until the HCG (pregnancy hormone levels in my blood) had returned to normal. It took until the end of March 2015 (five months after the initial operation) for my results to come back to normal. Every fortnight I posted the samples in a cardboard box and each time was reminded about my inability to procreate. I would call the hospital to get my results, hoping and praying that the numbers would keep dropping. Thankfully they did, albeit rather slowly. During that time we were not allowed to TTC. That was torture. All I wanted to do was get back to it and conceive again. I was just so desperate to have a baby. It was a long and anxious wait during which I felt very sorry for myself. It was around this time that I really began struggling to cope. My mental health was taking an absolute pounding.

ABOUT YOU

NO ONE is YOU...

...and that's YOUR SUPERPOWER

What are you good at?

_____

_____

_____

_____

What do you like about yourself?

_____

_____

_____

_____

What are you proud of your body for?

_____

_____

_____

_____

OTHER PEOPLE'S GOOD NEWS

Between December and March not a day went by when I didn't think about our situation, about being childless. We were childless and not allowed to do anything about it. I had my fortnightly tests done which were sent to Charing Cross Hospital and we just waited. We lived week to week; tests then results, tests then results. We were in limbo. Most days I would be fine and just distract myself with normal mundane things but other days it would creep up on me. Anything can trigger the tidal wave of emotions; feelings of bitterness, grief, guilt and failure. I call these the 'ugly' feelings. The sadness and jealousy was now accompanied by an undeniable feeling of embarrassment, I was embarrassed about not being able to do what everyone else could do.

It felt like everyone was having babies. I hated scrolling through my Facebook feed and seeing scan pictures. I couldn't stand hearing people talking about their pregnancy but worst of all was the face-to-face announcements. Several of my nearest and dearest had announced their pregnancies to us in person, usually with consideration, good intentions and acknowledgement of our difficulties. Despite this, it is still tough to deal with and in these situations I would just find myself not knowing what to say or how to act. My reactions and 'congratulations' would usually be really over the top as some kind of compensation for the obvious insincerity of it.

There was a turning point when I realised that I was not coping and needed to get some help. It came shortly after we had gotten the 'all clear' from Charing Cross Hospital and were given the go ahead to start TTC again. One Friday evening in April, around Easter time, I was headed out with some work friends and Scoop was giving me a lift. We had to swing by to collect my little sister as she was going too because she worked on the same ward at the time. She was still living with my mum so we popped in to say hi. When we went indoors my brother was there. This in itself was a real surprise as he and his wife had moved out to the Middle East with work in August the previous year just after getting married. We were not expecting him home, but there he was in my mum's living room with several other family members. Other than the fact that his visit was unexpected, there appeared to be something else going on that Scoop and I were not privy to. Everyone appeared to be very excitable and my mum ushered us to sit down on the sofa while they all surrounded us and watched our reaction as my brother told us that he and his wife were expecting a baby. In the next breath he added that it happened for them the first month they tried. That was like a dagger to my heart. I felt like he was saying, 'You know that thing you really want and have been trying so hard to get, well we've got it and we didn't even need to try.' This was followed by one of those silly hand flicks that rude boys do. I don't know why he did that; he isn't/wasn't ever a rude boy.

Some days the feelings creep up on you but there are other days when they come out of nowhere and you feel like you have been punched in the gut! Now, I have no idea what sort of a reaction everyone was expecting from us but they obviously hadn't predicted the one they got. My mum was in tears because she was so excited that she would 'finally' be getting her first grandchild. I remember her scanning my face for some happiness but there was none. She tried to get a positive reaction from me, 'Isn't it wonderful Laura?' she said. I was devastated and couldn't hide it. I was embarrassed because we weren't able to make a baby and I felt like our noses were being rubbed in it and everyone was laughing at us. Of course I know they weren't but I felt like the way it was announced to us clearly demonstrated that there was no way they understood our pain, not even my own family. It took everything I had to not simply break down in front of everyone. I understand that maybe I was very sensitive at the time, having just been given the all clear from the molar pregnancy and of course I was pleased to be having a niece or nephew soon but my heartbreak overshadowed this... immensely. I don't know why we couldn't have been told via text like I had always asked. I have two theories; we were close so maybe they thought that their happy news would not have this negative effect on us, or maybe they felt like they owed us a personal announcement because of all that we had been through. My brother did try to tell us a few days prior to this when Scoop and I were chatting to him on Skype. He started saying something and then just froze on the screen with his mouth open. He stopped talking but the picture and sound was still on so I knew the signal hadn't failed. After about 30 seconds he waffled something about the internet being shit and then said goodbye. The next time I saw him was in my mum's living room. I had mentioned to Scoop at the time that the Skype thing was weird and I even suggested that I thought he was being awkward because they were pregnant. I think Scoop put this down to my paranoia, it wasn't the first time I had jumped to this assumption about people but this time I was bloody right! Even if it seemed that the announcement was insensitive, they obviously had considered our feelings or else they wouldn't have called us on Skype that day planning to let us know before the rest of the family. I guess on the day everyone just got a bit carried away and excited. Sometimes our grief would put people in an impossible situation and it's only looking back now that I can see that. I would not want to be told but I would be angry if I was the only one that didn't know, for example. When they announced their second pregnancy my brother messaged Scoop. I was still sad but I was pleased for them. I was able to hide my sadness from everyone (apart from Scoop) but be genuinely happy when I actually spoke to them next. I am incredibly thankful for that.

I have recently discussed this all with my brother. I let him read this section of the book; mostly because it is about him but also because I was worried that he might feel like he has been portrayed as a bit of an arsehole. He did. When writing a memoir it is difficult to remain true to your experiences as well as being 100% true to the facts. This is because you are relying solely on your memory; the way that *you* felt and how *you* perceived a situation. What came out of our discussion was that he and his wife were incredibly nervous about telling us and they had indeed planned to tell us in a different way but due to circumstances and feeling the emotional enormity of the situation, they were unable to. In fact, the way we ended up being told came about due to a series of unplanned events that we were unaware of at the time and they felt terrible about this. Although I remember everyone seeming excitable, my brother assures me that in his case it was definitely more nervousness. And as for the funny hand flick, well maybe he did have a bit of rude boy phase back in the day and in his awkwardness it just slipped out.

I felt awful for not being able to congratulate them or be excited for them and I feel so guilty about this, even now. The night we were told the news I went out and got absolutely wasted, I just needed to forget about it. I wasn't ready to deal with it and luckily I was on a night out with nurses who are renowned for being animals! The following day I was incredibly hungover and it was probably the Tequila Rose that was to blame (I wonder if anyone actually drinks that stuff sober). My brother had stayed at our house that night. His wife was on her way down from visiting her family and she would be staying with us for a few days too. I love my brother and his wife dearly. They lived with us for two years prior to moving out to the Middle East and we got on very well. They are some of my most favourite people in the world and I would do anything for them but I could not face them that morning, even after not seeing them for eight months. I hid away in my bedroom, managing only a simple hello when my sister in law arrived. I blamed it on a headache but it was really my heart that was aching. When you hear other people's happy news it just brings home that deep sense of loss in your own life and exaggerates it tenfold.

This is when I sought help from a professional and was referred for counselling. It was all getting too much for me and I needed to find a way of coping with other people being pregnant. It was beginning to make me avoid people and situations. I was withdrawing from everyone around me and didn't like the bitter person I was becoming. I used to be the life and soul of a party, the organiser of events and the last-man-standing on a night out. I would never miss a social gathering, I had always enjoyed family time and loved being around children but this wasn't the case anymore. I felt awkward, paranoid and anxious. I would love to say that the counselling was really helpful but if I am honest it wasn't, but then again I didn't give it much of a chance. The counsellor kept trying to tell me that I needed to mourn the losses of the individual babies but it wasn't those individual beings that I grieved for. It's not like the grief that you have when you lose someone you love, who you know and have made memories with.

It's a grief for the hopes and dreams for the future and the memories that you never had the chance to make. It's a desperate longing to be a mum. That is what I grieved for, motherhood. I just so desperately wanted to be able to have a baby and I realised that the only way of getting through this was to be able to have one. The problem being that I had no idea when that would be or if it was even possible. So, in the meantime we needed a distraction; something to take our minds off of it all.

I needed some joy in my life, something nice to look forward to. Our lives were being taken over by sadness, bitterness and heartache. We had put our lives on hold because we thought we would have a baby soon but this wasn't turning out to be the case. I was almost 30 and was very down in the dumps because I wasn't content with my life. I didn't own a house, wasn't married and hadn't started our family. I always had this image of where I would be by the age of 30 and so far I was nowhere near it. We couldn't afford to buy a house and we clearly weren't having children any time soon, if ever, so I did some research and worked out that we could get married and it didn't actually need to cost a fortune like we had initially thought. In May, we did a contractual spit handshake and started planning our wedding for the following January. It was not the romantic proposal I had always dreamed of but that was okay. We were getting married and that was all that mattered. I then distracted myself with wedding planning and hoped that I would get pregnant in the meantime.

We started dieting and lost eight stone between us, three stone of that was mine. We had never been slim but in the past couple of years we had piled on the pounds. I have always been a comfort eater and we were a bad influence on each other, we still are in fact. We knew we needed to do it to optimise our health and therefore chances of having a baby but also so that we didn't look back on wedding pictures with regret. We continued to try to conceive for the rest of the year and everyone said that *it will happen* when you least expect it or when you stop trying so hard. We thought that focusing on the wedding might help with this but of course it didn't. We didn't fall pregnant once in 2015, but that was okay because at least there was something to look forward to. It made Christmas a bit easier in one respect that year; however, devastating family circumstances meant that it was a terribly sad time too. I'll come on to this later.

Now I know that I have put a lot of emphasis on Christmas but that is because it is my favourite time of year, or at least it used to be. I used to love Christmas. I guess it stems from having a younger sister. My brother and I were just reaching the stage of doubting if the big man in the red suit really existed when our little sister came along and the magic was brought back to life again. My brother and I milked it a bit and the excitement of Christmas was prolonged for a few more years. The festive season had become a really difficult time for us over the previous few years. After all, Christmas is for children. The excitement and magic for all the little people in the world is what it is all about. However, Christmas 2015 had a different focus. We looked forward to the wedding in January and we tried not to put too much weight back on!

Another time of year that I found terribly difficult was Mother's Day. This was a sad and lonely day for several years. For me, Mother's Day is a reminder of what is missing from our lives. That big gaping hole. The missing piece of our jigsaw. The sense of loss is real. It is deep, heart wrenching and real! Each year I would wonder if the next year would be the one when I joined the mummy club that seemed to rapidly grow among my group of friends and family. I just felt so left out and desperately wanted to be a part of it. We needed a distraction from the baby making and the wedding would do just that, we hoped.

The other focus for us in 2015 that helped distract us from our childlessness was all the testing we went through following the third pregnancy loss. Not only was there the testing for the molar pregnancy but the NHS also did investigations into possible causes of miscarriages. It is standard practice to start this only after someone has experienced three miscarriages. It seems horrible that someone should have to go through so many miscarriages to be able to have testing done but the policies are dictated by funding. The area of miscarriage is largely underfunded and poorly understood due to limited research in the area. All too often the cause of miscarriage is attributed to just 'bad luck'. Tommy's, the baby charity, started the 'Tell Me Why' campaign in 2019 to help give answers to parents who go through pregnancy loss and stillbirth. One or two miscarriages are sadly rather common; 25% of all pregnancies end in miscarriage. However, it is as few as one in every 100 women who experience recurrent miscarriages of three or more in a row. The cause of these recurrent pregnancy losses is unknown in about half of the cases. The main issues are chromosomal abnormalities, hormone imbalance, blood clotting disorders, uterine problems or cervical weakness. (Tommy's, 2019; Tommy's, 2020)

Our testing would hopefully rule some of these things out and the best-case scenario was that we would find a treatable cause. It was a nervy time having the testing done but I felt that at least something was being done. We were being proactive finally and that felt good.

The first line of testing at the recurrent miscarriage clinic involved a lot of blood tests and a 4D scan of the uterus. The blood results were borderline for a blood clotting disorder APS (antiphospholipid syndrome), commonly known as 'sticky blood' so I was advised to take aspirin and use blood thinning injections for future pregnancies. I was told that the sticky blood would prevent the placenta from forming properly thus not transporting vital nutrients to the baby, resulting in an unsustainable pregnancy. The 4D scan showed an abnormality too. I may need an operation on my uterus as they could see what they thought was a septum. This is known as a 'heart shaped womb'. It looked like a partial septum, which would not have a blood flow to it. That meant if a pregnancy was to implant on the septum, it would fail for this reason. The scan also showed some 'abnormal masses' in the left ovary so I had further tests to rule out cancer. These were probably formalities and them being over cautious but I was scared. In a way, I sort of wanted something to be wrong because at least we could try and sort it out but talk of cancer (again) was terribly scary. Thankfully, the tests on the ovary came back normal. I could have an operation on the abnormal uterus and I could take medications for the blood clotting disorder. I felt like we were getting somewhere. We had answers and a treatment plan. It was such a relief that a cause was found and it could be treated.

However, this relief was short-lived. I went on to have a second set of blood tests six weeks later due to the first ones showing a borderline result. I also had a scan of my kidneys because uterine abnormalities are commonly associated with abnormal kidneys. My kidneys were fine. The second set of blood tests were normal and following a second (pre-operation) 4D scan of the uterus, it was concluded that I did not actually have a septum so the surgery was cancelled. So, I now felt like we were getting nowhere! It appeared that there was nothing wrong with me and it was all just 'bad luck'. I wondered how everything could be so uncertain and our plan of action change so much in a matter of weeks. In fact, now there was no plan of action at all. Testing was not required for Scoop because we were able to fall pregnant. We were told there was nothing wrong with either of us and we should just try again. Due to being able to fall pregnant we were not able to be referred for fertility tests and would not be entitled to IVF or the like. The only change they suggested was that I continue on the aspirin for any future pregnancies. It seemed to be a common drug that people took following miscarriages and it was unlikely to do me any harm, so it was worth a try. That was the extent of our treatment plan after all the testing. So that was it then, back to baby making and hopefully the aspirin would solve all of our problems. I tried to remain optimistic about it all because really I had no other option, but I knew deep down that our problem was not just bad luck. I was so scared of not getting pregnant but equally petrified of actually getting pregnant because I feared the same thing happening again.

ABOUT YOU

Suggestions for marking your loss,

* Document your memories, hopes, fears and feelings for that pregnancy in a book or memory box.
* Plant a tree or flower in your garden.
* Light a candle on anniversaries. Join the wave of light in Baby Loss Awareness Week (9th-15th October).
* Make a donation to charity or do a sponsored event like a 5k run.

There are lots of lovely ways to remember your babies. How have you commemorated your loss(es)?

_____

_____

_____

_____

_____

_____

_____

_____

_____

FIGHTING FOR ANSWERS

We got married on 30th January in 2016. Before I tell you about it though, I feel that I should mention the proposal. I have already said that when we 'agreed' to get married it was with a spit handshake in the previous May. I wondered if Scoop would actually get me an engagement ring and propose to me properly. As the predictable opportunities came and went (my birthday in June, Christmas, New Year's Eve) I assumed and hoped that he would propose to me on our wedding day in front of everyone, after I had walked down the aisle. I imagined it to be ever so romantic. In my imagination I walked down the aisle and Scoop would ask the registrar if he could interrupt before we started the ceremony. That is when he would get down on one knee and propose. There were no other significant dates between the 1st January and the wedding at the end of the month so it made perfect sense. However, what actually happened was a bit different. I was at work on the ward on a night shift, my last shift before I had time off for the wedding. It was the 20th January. I was the nurse in charge of the unit so was based at the nurses' station and coordinating the shift. This involved constant phone calls to and from the doctors, A&E staff, site managers and the wards as well as helping out the staff on shifts with caring for patients where required. I hoped for a non-eventful and quiet last shift before my few weeks of annual leave where I would go and get hitched. When one of my colleagues came rushing down the ward, hastily asking for my assistance with a poorly patient in bed four, I rushed to help her. As we ran up the ward I remember thinking that I was pretty certain that bed four was empty so assumed that in her fluster she had said the wrong bed number. To be honest the fact that my colleague who never went anywhere fast was actually running up the ward, was pretty distracting. When we arrived into the bay the curtain was drawn round the bed. I pulled it open to find Scoop on one knee with a ring in his hand. Ten days before our wedding he asked me to marry him and of course I said yes, after calling him a 'dick'. The patient in the bed opposite (bed three) starting clapping and cheering, I think it made her evening. She was telling her family about it in the morning but I don't think they believed her, just thought she was getting muddled and confused. My colleagues and my sister were all gathered in the bay to witness it too. It was very sweet and a bit of a relief to be turning up to my wedding with an engagement ring.

There was one thing that I hoped would not arrive in time for the wedding and that was Aunt Flo. The day before the wedding, we went to drop to some things off at the venue in Tunbridge Wells. It was all very exciting and the barn looked ever so romantic with the crisp white table cloths, candelabras and twinkly fairy lights. I couldn't wait for it to be tomorrow already. We said goodbye to the boys as they were staying to set up the venue. They were then having a last hoorah before the big day and staying in the hotel that night. I gave Scoop a big squeeze and a smooch before I headed back home with the girls. We were having our hair done at my mum's house that evening and I was staying over there. I had a lingering headache all day long and just assumed it was stress but by the time I was sat down having my hair done, it was absolutely throbbing. I suffer quite badly with migraines so was terrified that this would develop into one. I took some tablets and crossed my fingers because I knew all too well that if this was a migraine I was in for a horrific night and would struggle to function properly the next day. Fortunately it wasn't a migraine but it was good old Aunty Florence that was causing my banging headache. Aunt Flo had arrived five days early. What the hell was she doing here? Of all the times that you don't want your period to come unexpectedly, your wedding has to be top of the list. This is of course followed closely by holidays, swimming, a third date and generally any time you are planning on wearing something white. I mean periods are tedious at the best of times and you really begin to hate them when they mean that you still aren't pregnant but on the wedding day too, it's just a pain in the arse. Having said that, as soon as the red river started flowing the headache improved. Or maybe it was just the prosecco that did that.

Our wedding day was perfect. Surprisingly the sun was shining all day, which was wonderful. It was a real bonus. Having gone for a wedding in the winter months because it was a lot cheaper, we were so lucky that we ended up with better weather than some of the summer weddings we have been to. It is such a special feeling being surrounded by all your family and friends. There aren't many times in your life when you will have all your favourite people in one room so I made sure to take it all in. My brother, his wife and my new baby niece flew home from the Middle East for the wedding and it was wonderful to have them there and to meet the new addition. I was so excited to meet her and of course I loved her without question from the second she entered this world. I was so sad when we had to say goodbye to them after a few days. The jealousy and resentment that I feel towards pregnant couples has always only ever lasted until the baby is born at which point I become besotted and can't get enough of the new-born snuggles. I just seem to have problems dealing with pregnant women. I am not entirely sure why this is and there is nothing that I can do to control these feelings, trust me I have tried, but it has been an ongoing pattern since the ugly feelings began.

After the wedding, we took our beloved dog Cooper away with us for the week to a cottage in Suffolk. Cooper is the apple of Scoop's eye; he loves him so much. Once I asked him if he actually loved the dog more than he loved me, to which his response was that he loved us both the same! THE SAME! The cheek of it! Cooper has inevitably become our saving grace over the years, it's like having our very own little therapy dog. In fact, after each loss we've been through (and in some cases during it), we have gone to the same woods and walked the same route with Cooper. There is something comforting about that walk. Even now, when I am there I feel sort of connected to all the babies that I never got to meet. It truly is a special place to me.

We had a lovely time on our mini-moon. We looked around antique shops, visited village tea rooms, had a day at a beautiful spa and went on lots of muddy dog walks. We felt so relaxed afterwards but before we knew it we were back to the daily grind in the middle of winter. What a come down that was after a few weeks off for the wedding and our trip away. However, mundane life carried on for only a few weeks and it didn't take long for us to find out we were pregnant again. When we found out, it felt like it was just meant to be. I couldn't believe that we had spent all that time in the lead up to our wedding TTC but now we were married it seemed to happen straight away. Was someone looking down on us? I'm not sure about my beliefs regarding a big man in the sky but it somehow seemed that now we were married it was legal and proper and okay for us to be having a baby. It made me rather optimistic but it all ended quite abruptly with a fourth miscarriage only a week or so after getting the BFP. It was a spontaneous miscarriage. I had a scan and everything had come away. This is what is known as a chemical pregnancy. It is where a pregnancy ends before five weeks, usually shortly after the implantation of the embryo into the lining of the uterus and often due to chromosomal abnormality. It shows up as a faint positive on a pregnancy test which will often fade or disappear in any subsequent tests. Those two lines on the test trigger a tidal wave of excitement and emotions which comes crashing down with that first spot of blood. I barely had any time off work following this, I didn't want to be sat at home dwelling on it. We fell pregnant again on the following cycle, once again taking advantage of the increased fertility following a miscarriage but I started bleeding during those early weeks. It was looking like this would be our fifth miscarriage but I needed to wait a week for another scan to assess the viability, in case I'd got my dates wrong or my cycle length was skewed by the last miscarriage.

I felt like such a fool for even believing that it might happen for us. Stupidly I thought that now we were married, had lost weight and had been taking the aspirin that things might be different this time. I was so hopeful but incredibly naive to think that it would actually work for us. I was taking extra medication in the form of progesterone suppositories to make my womb more 'habitable'. These little greasy bullets that I had to insert into my back passage every night were absolutely wonderful. *Note the sarcasm.* The evidence for them preventing miscarriage was not overwhelming. There had been some success in small studies that suggest benefits and we knew that it was unlikely to cause harm so it was worth a shot but oh my goodness; the side effects. Not only do you have an oily discharge from you back passage (or vagina dependent on where you choose to insert it - FYI it's less leaky from the bum hole), you also have to deal with side effects of sore boobs, abdominal cramping, nausea, fatigue, bloating, fluctuating emotions and irritability. Does this sound familiar? It reeks of pregnancy symptoms again doesn't it! It's so cruel!

A week later that second scan showed that the pregnancy was not viable as it had not progressed in that time. I had a decision to make. I could either wait for the pregnancy to come away by itself, take medications to help speed up this process or have an operation to remove the products, like I had done before. I opted for the operation for two reasons. I didn't want this torture drawn out and I had heard some horror stories about medical management. I wanted it over and done with as soon as possible so I could move on and try again. I also wanted to have the products tested again, in case there was a clue as to why this kept happening. I'd had enough of this and I wanted answers. I had the Surgical Management of Miscarriage and was just as emotional after this one as I was with the previous operation. My physical recovery was okay but emotionally and mentally it was taking its toll and I needed more time off work to cope with this. What a terrible start to married life; two miscarriages within a few months of us saying 'I do'. I felt so low. What had we done to deserve this? I couldn't help but wonder if I would ever have a baby and I felt so guilty that poor Scoop was married to me now. He might never have the chance to be a daddy. I used to have nightmares that he left me and had a baby with someone else. It broke my heart that I couldn't give him what he wanted. I told him about these nightmares and initially he told me I was being silly and tried to reassure me but he did get angry when they kept happening. He said I acted resentful towards him for something that was happening in my head when I was sleeping. I carried on having the dreams for some time after this; I just stopped telling him about them.

The results of the testing came back six weeks later and showed that the pregnancy tested normal. There was nothing wrong with it. The scan results were also normal. They found no reason as to why the pregnancy failed. This got me thinking, as I had always thought that our bad luck was caused by my (what I assumed were) less than optimal eggs. I imagined that the bad eggs when fertilised were creating embryos that were incompatible with life meaning that the pregnancy had no chance of progressing and we would just have to wait for the time when we had a good egg that fertilised. However, the test results that came back suggested otherwise. This was a normal embryo so why had the pregnancy failed? It was obviously my fault. I started doing some research into other common causes of miscarriages that would fit this theory. I ended up doing research into autoimmune factors in pregnancy.

After some research, I came to the conclusion that my body was rejecting perfectly normal embryos, treating them as a foreign object. I have a relatively minor skin condition, but it is autoimmune related, so as far as I was concerned this seemed like a pretty sensible conclusion to arrive at, considering all the other tests had been normal. The treatment for this is simply medication. The only problem was that the testing is not funded by the NHS at my local trust. I asked the hospital consultant about this and reluctantly they made a referral to someone more specialist at another local hospital.

In the meantime I was also booked in for a HSG scan (hysterosalpingography) which involves having dye flushed through the cervix and into the uterus and fallopian tubes. The procedure is done under x-ray so that images can be taken to see if there are any blockages in the tubes.

I waited for the appointment with the specialist in June. I was so relieved to finally be going to see them because I felt like something good would come of it; I might finally get some answers and get the appropriate treatment. I could not have been more wrong. I was so disappointed. It was awful. The doctor was terribly condescending and dismissive. He started the consultation with, 'So, tell me what you understand a miscarriage to be'. I was gob smacked really, I must have looked like an idiot, I didn't know what to say. I toyed with the idea of telling him that I was a nurse but I didn't. I'm not sure why but I doubt it would have changed the outcome of the consultation anyway. One by one he suggested that I be started on several different medications, all of which I had already tried and still miscarried. When I informed him of this he sighed and explained that it was probably 'just bad luck'. He told me that I was still young so I should keep trying and I could come back to see him when I was 32 if I had not had a baby by then. That was a year away at this point. I was so upset and frustrated by this. It seemed so easy for them to just attribute it to bad luck and this explanation is accepted by many women, but I wasn't having it. I asked him about the research I had done about autoimmune conditions and the treatment that I understood may be beneficial but he chuckled and shut me down. Was this really happening to me? He didn't think I needed the medication and couldn't do the tests anyway as they were too specialist. With regards to the results of the HSG, his response was, 'Oh yeah, that was normal'. It just felt like a pointless exercise attending this appointment which I had held out so much hope for. I walked away not knowing what to do next. I felt like he had not listened to my concerns or even pretended to be interested. I was incredibly disheartened as this consultant was meant to be the most specialist in the area. I got in the car and I broke down in tears. I was in too much of a state to even call Scoop to tell him what had happened. I was in disbelief and had lost all hope. I did not know where to turn. I didn't think I would ever have a baby and I felt like no-one gave a shit! What the hell was I going to do now? It took me so long to gather myself that when I finally started the car up to drive home, I couldn't get through the barrier because I had taken too long since paying and my ticket had expired.

Five miscarriages could not be just bad luck. I started seeking advice from the online community. Oh my! What a community! There are thousands of women from all over the world who are dealing with recurrent pregnancy loss. I am so thankful to this community for all the support and guidance I have received over the years. These women have been through it and we understand each other. It is a safe space for us to vent and moan to strangers about our real-life problems. Obviously, you have to find the right group(s) to suit you but generally there is no judgment or bitchiness, just genuine support and understanding. They are also great for offering advice. These warrior women are empowered and incredibly knowledgeable and it was here that another specialist was recommended to me. I had heard of this professor before as I had a friend who had been on a similar journey to me and had been to this clinic. She was successfully carrying twins at this time so something must have gone right for her. I begged my GP to refer me out of the local area to see this specialist, at St Mary's Hospital in Paddington, London. After a long debate and discussion they agreed and made the referral. I was glad I had done my research before making that call as I really had to fight to be heard. Once again I was hopeful that we would get answers. I was positive that this third specialist would have some answers for me, like she did for my friend. During the time that I waited for this appointment I changed jobs. I had always worried about changing jobs due to the fear of not being eligible for maternity pay when I fell pregnant. However, I couldn't hold on to a pregnancy, the job was becoming too stressful and I wanted to get out of there so I bit the bullet and left. In fact over the years a lot of things were put on hold. We avoided booking holidays, planning renovations etc because I always planned I would be pregnant.

I went from stressful shift work to a Monday to Friday job, working normal office hours. It was still working within nursing, but it was assessment based as opposed to in an acute hospital setting. There was still pressure (I mean what job doesn't have pressure?) but it was otherwise less stressful and easier on the mind and body. The training for the job involved me working in sunny Stoke-on-Trent for five weeks, during which time we missed two periods of ovulation. Typical. Aside from that we had some lovely trips away in 2016. We went to Glastonbury festival (a first for me as this was another thing we had always put off due to pregnancy plans) and we had a fantastic honeymoon in Tuscany. It was an amazing holiday and so relaxing; we stayed at an adult-only hotel. I always tried to focus on the benefits of being childless; lots of holidays, weekend lie-ins, not having to pay for childcare, being able to spontaneously go out together etc. I had to remind myself of the perks. There are many and it helps to remind yourself of them when struggling with fertility and pregnancy loss, however being childless not by choice is absolutely infuriating.

When my care was transferred to the recurrent miscarriage specialist in London towards the end of the year, they did all of the same tests that the first specialist had done. They found out that I actually did have a heart shaped womb as previously suspected. I was told that it was unlikely to be the direct cause for our losses but if I was ever to carry further in the pregnancy, this septum was likely to cause problems in the latter stages. I was booked in for an operation the following March, in 2017, and couldn't believe that this was happening now when I could have had the operation done almost two years prior. I was told not to conceive while waiting for this. So, we were five miscarriages down and there was still no real known cause for them. While we waited for the operation which probably wouldn't make any difference to our chances of becoming parents, so many of our family and friends we're starting, growing and even finishing making their families. I really struggled with this because I felt like everyone else was getting what they wanted and we were just stuck in the same position, getting nowhere and running out of time. I could feel my body clock ticking.

In March 2017 I got the train to London on my own very early in the morning for the operation. I was having a hysteroscopy, which is where they look inside the uterus. Once inside they would assess the situation. I had consented for them to remove a septum and anything else that may cause problems with future pregnancies. It transpired that I did have a septum and it was 'much more significant' than they had initially thought. That was removed along with a polyp. I had two coils inserted and was discharged the same day with HRT tablets. If I remember correctly, the coils are to prevent adhesions in the uterus and the HRT is to promote blood flow to the area to aide healing, I think. If I'm completely honest I was rather jaded when the registrar was talking me through all of this following the surgery.

Scoop got the train up to meet me so he could escort me home. St Mary's Hospital in Paddington is a very old hospital and the buildings are like mazes. We ended up walking down three or four flights of stairs as we couldn't find the lift. I could feel myself bleeding heavily as I walked. By the time we reached Paddington train station I felt faint and my vision went blurry. I sat on the floor outside the train station and gathered myself. We ate a Burger King (any excuse) and then slowly made our way home. Recovery from this operation was longer than I had anticipated but I guess the septum was larger than they had anticipated too. At my six-week check-up they removed the two coils that had been fitted. I still had some pain but was told that it was normal so was discharged from this clinic and advised to try again.

Despite not having much faith in my body but at a loss as to what else to do, we did just that. We tried again.

It took six months to fall pregnant again. We had another early miscarriage in the September. I got my BFP on the Friday and by the Monday morning I was bleeding. I had let myself get excited, again. I felt so stupid but when it is everything you have ever wanted you can't help it. When I started bleeding, I knew it was doomed. I went to work and carried on for the whole week as if nothing had happened. What else could I do? There was no point going to the EPU, they couldn't save the pregnancy. All they could do was confirm my fears, but I already knew. I was becoming a bit of an expert at miscarrying but that isn't something you want on your CV.

I had become disconnected from the pregnancies themselves. I no longer thought of the pregnancy as a baby and I didn't mourn the loss of a little being. I understand how harsh this must sound but I promised myself I would be completely open and honest when writing about my experiences. Looking back now I can see that this is an act self-preservation and a self-defence mechanism. I wasn't hurting because an embryo didn't develop into a foetus or a foetus didn't develop into a baby. What was hurting me the most during these times was the thought of my life without any babies. I was grieving for the loss of motherhood. I desperately longed to be a mummy and it made my heart ache that this wasn't looking like it would be possible. My heart physically hurt. I had lost all hope that it would ever happen for us and although I had become quite depressed over the years it was noticeable now more than ever. I was feeling under pressure to enjoy myself when all I wanted to do was hibernate. I found myself in that all too familiar situation of 'what next?' I couldn't keep doing this, it was driving me insane and started to take its toll on my mental health and subsequently on our relationship. I had become a very sad person and I rarely found joy in anything.

It must have been so hard to be around me when I was going through this.

Once again, I went back online and reached out for help from those complete strangers who understood me so well. It is truly amazing how these women who you have never met can provide more support to you than your nearest and dearest but I guess it is because they just 'get it'. The recurrent pregnancy loss and miscarriage communities online are true warriors and they know their stuff. I had sought advice before but this time I poured my heart out. Instead of asking a simple question or seeking a bit of advice I started from the very beginning of my journey. I typed about what had happened over the years; the losses, the tests, the specialists, the results, and I wrote about how I felt at a loss about what to do next. I wrote about it all. I was almost ready to give up on having a baby and this was my last ditch attempt to seek advice and I made that very clear in my posts on different forums. Maybe these women knew something that I didn't. I was astounded by the responses I received. There were messages of support, advice, sadness, empathy and most importantly messages of hope. This was important to me because it was something I was seriously lacking in. I kept hearing the same consultant's name over and over. Many people were suggesting I get referred to one particular doctor, a reproductive immunologist at Epsom Hospital. Once again I did my research and begged my GP for another referral. I think that being a health professional myself helped with getting my voice heard and referrals made when I requested them. I am thankful for this, but I worry about others who are fighting for answers too. I wonder if they would be as persistent and have as much luck with their requests. I really hope so. If I had not taken matters into my own hands by researching and requesting referrals, I have no doubt that my journey would have been very different indeed.

If it was an autoimmune problem that I had then this was the doctor who would be able to find out and treat me accordingly. When I received my appointment it was six months away. That is how busy he was. I was told by his secretary when I contacted them that he was the only specialist in the UK at the time that was doing such tests on the NHS, elsewhere you had to pay privately to have them done. This was why the waiting list was so long. I was prepared to pay anything if it meant I could have a baby, but I was all too aware that there was a possibility that the tests could come back saying that there was nothing wrong. For the sake of six months I wasn't sure I could justify spending all our money and getting into more debt. The longer it took me to decide, the closer the appointment got. We reached a point when it became a no brainer to just wait for the NHS appointment. I hoped it would be worth the wait but I doubted it. I had become a bit of a pessimist. In the meantime, more and more people were getting pregnant, even the people who had previously struggled and I had looked to for support. I felt so alone in my real life. I kept hearing the same old words from people. 'It will happen,' they'd say but I just didn't think it would anymore. The only place I felt like people understood me was on a Facebook group full of strangers and what wonderful strangers they are.

ABOUT YOU

The NHS currently commences standard testing after 3 miscarriages. Below are the baseline tests. Further testing may be required depending on these initial results. There is space for you to jot down your results.

Karyotyping ( ) Foetal/Parental
The foetus is tested for chromosomal abnormalities and if a genetic abnormality is found then you and your partner may have DNA test and dependent on the results you may be referred for genetic counseling.

_____
_____
_____

Ultrasound Scan ( )
A transvaginal ultrasound and a 3D scan will be done to check the structure of your womb, ovaries and fallopian tubes for any abnormalities.

_____
_____
_____

Blood Tests
Clotting:
Lupus Antocoagulant ( )
Anticardiolipin Antibodies ( )

_____
_____
_____

Hormonal:
Luteinising Hormone ( )
Thyroid Panel ( )

Hysterosalpingogram (HSG) ( )
You may also be offered this scan where an image is taken when dye is injected into the uterus. It will show up any abnormalities in the shape of the uterus and any blockages in the fallopian tubes

With a history of recurrent miscarriages most EPU's will offer an early reassurance ultrasound scan in further pregnancies.

It is important to realise that there may be a combination of causes leading to miscarriage, rather than a single underlying one. However investigations may not identify any specific cause or causes in the majority of cases. Remember that statistics show that you are more likely to have a successful pregnancy next time than to miscarry again.

(NHS, 2018)

DEALING WITH CONFLICTING EMOTIONS

At the end of 2017 I reached the end of my tether. I was so fed up with it. I worked out that I had been pregnant for nine months in total. We had no living children and had been through six pregnancy losses. Waiting so long for our dream to come true was becoming increasingly hard. It was made more difficult knowing that what I was dreaming of was coming so easily to so many others. I was constantly reminded of my failure to create a baby to start the family that we both longed for.

Over the years that we had been dealing with these losses, I felt like I was stabbed in the heart on a regular basis. My heart hurt, it physically hurt. I know couples who met and had a child and those who had had two children in the time that we had been trying for our family. I know children who had birthdays on our due dates. I couldn't help but wonder how different things could have been. I was now at the point where every single pregnancy announcement hurt me. Be it celebrities, colleagues, friends, Facebook friends and even friends of friends that I had never even met. That is not to say that I was not happy for these women, I truly was, it just reminded me of our incredibly sad and hopeless situation. I often pondered... Why me? Why us? What is wrong with me? Why has it happened so many bloody times?

If I'm honest, really honest, it's jealousy. Why them? What have they done differently? How did it happen so easily for them? I'd have given anything to be in their position. With every loss we experienced, I had a deeper feeling of grief. It doesn't get easier. But it does get easier to make it look like it gets easier.

Recurrent pregnancy loss changes the person you are. It changes your outlook on everything but particularly on pregnancy itself. It changes the way you see people and even the way you see the world. People take it for granted and assume that it will just happen for them, after all it should be so easy, right? Not for me and not for many others. When I think about pregnancy, it brings fear, anxiety, doubt and an overwhelming feeling of hopelessness. I resented feeling like this and resented the inability to ever feel the joy of pregnancy that so many others do. Recurrent pregnancy loss had taken over my life and was my main focus for over five years. It was terribly exhausting to feel so sad for so long. I considered myself a strong person and I was quite good at pretending everything was fine, however it was becoming increasingly difficult and tiring. I dealt with it by avoiding situations where I knew I would have to put my 'game face' on. It was easier to just be by myself and stay at home. I was aware that this was not healthy, but for me it was about self-preservation. In contrast Scoop just wanted to forget about our struggles and coped with this by focusing on his rugby and spending time with friends. I can't blame him, I wasn't much fun to be around at this time. Recurrent pregnancy loss impacted on my relationships with so many people. It knocked my confidence and impaired my ability, drive and ambition in everyday life. I became less productive and less motivated, at work and at home. I just couldn't be bothered. It was a dark and lonely place to be. I didn't even recognise the person I had become over the previous five years and this change was permanent. I was still able to put my 'game face' on but it happened less often and was probably less convincing. The trauma of recurrent pregnancy loss cannot be erased. Those six pregnancy losses I experienced had changed me, forever. A recent study by Tommy's showed that women may be at risk of post-traumatic stress disorder following early pregnancy losses (Tommy's, 2020). The results of this research were not known at the time I was going through this all but it certainly explains a lot.

I felt guilty about my lack of interest and excitement about other people's pregnancies, even those very close to me. I tried so hard not to feel resentment and envy and I know that people try to be understanding and supportive, but I just felt so lonely. I felt like no one actually understood. But how could they? They had not been through it themselves. People who had experienced a miscarriage before having a baby would reach out to me and tell me that they understood how I felt and that our next pregnancy would 'the one'. I don't doubt that their experience was devastating but it wasn't the same as mine and I didn't want people to compare their experiences with mine as it was almost as if they were minimising my grief. I wasn't interested in anyone else's heartbreak because mine was all consuming. Poor Scoop had to listen to me crying myself to sleep at night and witness me randomly welling up or sobbing for what appeared to be no reason at all. I know he was suffering too and he felt so bad that he could not make things better for me, for us.

We so desperately wanted to have a family but at the end of 2017 we found ourselves at the point where the idea of having our own baby was impossible. How long would we carry on doing this? We couldn't keep trying to get pregnant if we knew it would end in loss, that was just silly, and it wasn't fair to keep putting ourselves or the people around us through that. Those familiar feelings of failure were rising, and my desire to be a mum was as strong as it had always been. I so wanted to make Scoop into a daddy and give our parents another grandchild. I truly felt like it is what I was put on this earth to do. I couldn't even do that and it made me feel like a failure. So, we looked into adoption and both felt that it was something we were interested in. We knew we had the appointment with the specialist at Epsom in April but we weren't convinced this would solve our problems so in the meantime we decided to get the ball rolling in the long and complex adoption process.

In early December we attended an open evening. We arrived flustered as we were late because it was chucking it down, traffic had been terrible and then I took a wrong turn. It had caused us to bicker on the hurried and wet walk to the council building where the meeting was being held. Tensions were running high. I knew that Scoop would rather not have been there, he didn't want to admit defeat as he was still so positive that we would be able to have our own baby one day. I thought he was deluded and insisted he come along, even if it was just to humour me. He obliged. The room where the information evening was held was dark and gloomy and covered from floor to ceiling in varnished wood panelling. There were several other couples there who we eyed up as we helped ourselves to a cup of tea. I couldn't help but wonder what their stories were and why or how we had come to end up in the same room that evening.

Following the presentation from the social workers a woman who had successfully adopted the previous year talked us through the process. It all seemed quite smooth running for her, but I was aware that this wasn't always the case. Despite this we left the meeting feeling positive about the future and we started to imagine ourselves with children, with a family. I was ready to go for this full throttle. The sooner we got started the sooner we would have our babies. I was so excited and it was all I could talk about on the 20-minute drive home. I wanted to opt for siblings because that would mean not only would we keep a family together, but we would also create our own in one fell swoop. As soon as we got home, I started filling out the form. It was all fine until I got to the section where you have to confirm that you stopped trying to conceive more than six months ago. This wasn't the case for us; my last miscarriage was only a few months prior and I had no intention of stopping TTC. I actually considered lying but worried that it would impair our chances if we got found out. Scoop and I talked through our options, but it made complete sense why this policy was in place and we decided to respect it. They want you to have dealt with the grief and loss you have been through, and they want you to be fully committed to the adoption process. There, with my pen in hand hovering over the form, I realised I was not quite ready to let go of our dream of having a baby ourselves. I wasn't ready to close that door. Though our emotional energy reserves were low, and the thought of putting ourselves through it all again was painful, there was still a glimmer of light behind that door. We put adoption on the back burner and pinned all our hopes on our April appointment with the specialist in Epsom. In the meantime, we had to get through another childless Christmas.

Christmas was okay I guess. My brother, pregnant sister-in-law and niece were home for the festivities and it was so nice to have everyone together. I coped as I usually did by drinking a lot of fizzy shit and being my over-the-top, gregarious self. That is until about 8pm that night when it all got on top of me and I had a little silent cry in the corner. Scoop recognised that I had reached my limit of family time and baby talk and made our excuses so we could head home to put on pjs and eat chocolate.

My lovely nan turned 90 on New Year's Eve so we had a legendary family party at my uncle's house. My cousin's wife was pregnant too so her and my sister-in-law chatted about babies and everyone joined in the conversations. I was bitter, jealous and couldn't be around these conversations. I'm making myself sound crazy here but that's how I felt at the time, so paranoid and resentful. I mean why shouldn't they be allowed to be pregnant and talk about it with their family? I really was in a bad place. It was clear that getting smashed was my way of dealing with everything and it is safe to say that I over did it on the gin. From what I remember it was a very fun night in the end. It always is with my family! I suffered the consequences and required a few days off work to nurse my hangover. It must have been so obvious to work but I said I had diarrhoea and vomiting which enabled me to have a few days off, after all I was still vomiting so it was half true. I still felt rough when I went back to work, but it was the sore boobs that made me consider doing a pregnancy test. It was only bloody positive. It was a strong positive from the second I peed on the stick. There was none of the usual long three-minute wait and no need to squint or look at the test in a different light or from a different angle or use a different filter. For the first time ever, it was an instant strong positive. I worked out that this made me three weeks and four days pregnant, which also meant that I was pregnant when I consumed a gallon of gin on New Year's Eve. Oops (again). When I showed Scoop the positive test, he rolled his eyes. I laughed and said, "Here we go again - let's see how long this one lasts..."

I had the usual anxieties that follow a positive test. They seemed to get worse with every loss we endured. I have a fear that comes with every trip to the toilet, just in case I see blood on the tissue paper, like I did with that first miscarriage. I constantly feel my boobs to check they are still sore (so much so that I think I actually make them sore) and I hope and pray that I will wake up feeling sick in the morning. While I obsessed over symptoms, Scoop tried his best to forget that we were even pregnant. It's his way of protecting his emotions. Not acknowledging it and not getting excited about it makes any loss easier for him to deal with. I can't blame him for his defensive ways, in fact I wish I could switch off and forget about it too, at least until the second trimester. However, the heartburn, fatigue and giant tingly nipples prevent this from being possible. Instead I go from feeling excited to feeling anxious, dependent on the severity of symptoms that I experience on any given day.

Time goes so slowly in early pregnancy and I find myself wishing the days away. The due date of 16th September seemed so far away! Funnily enough one of my loveliest friends, who was also a colleague at the time, was due on the very same day. She had just started trying for a baby and I was so pleased that it happened for her so quickly. I wouldn't wish all that we had been through on my worst enemy, let alone one of my friends. In the very early days when we first discovered that we were both due at the same time, there was initial excitement however for me this soon faded. I realised that like everyone else who had ever gone on to have a baby while I had lost mine during the early stages, this would probably cause distance in our friendship and I was likely to resent her and feel terribly jealous of her pregnancy. Of course I hoped that this would not be the case at all and we talked about being on maternity leave together and taking our babies to the beach together in the summer, but I couldn't help but doubt if that would actually happen.

I had worked out that I would reach 12 weeks the week before Mother's Day. I planned to keep the pregnancy under wraps until 13 weeks to surprise our mums then. I know all our families have found our situation very tough to deal with and I would have loved to give them some good news for a change. I had been looking at 'grandma' Mother's Day gifts. I thought that it would be lovely to surprise them when we had reached a safer place in the pregnancy, when the risks of loss are lower. We would even have a scan picture by then. In the six previous pregnancies I had never got a scan picture. I'd had about 20 scans but never took away a picture. Not one. Ever. I really thought that this time was going to be different. This was our seventh pregnancy and I felt like we were owed some good luck. Everything felt positive. I kept telling myself that this pregnancy was going to be our lucky number seven, our rainbow after the storm.

The term for a healthy baby born following the heartbreak of miscarriage, pregnancy loss, stillbirth or neonatal death is 'rainbow baby'. This is because it signifies brightness, hope and beauty after something so scary and dark. I really like the sentiment and symbolism. However, you'll be well aware that rainbows don't always appear after storms. Sometimes there is a storm, the clouds clear slightly and then another storm comes rolling in.

In actual fact, it turned out to be our very Unlucky number seven. I started spotting at five weeks and six days. We were away for the weekend, staying with family down in Somerset. I tried to ignore it and carry on as usual and enjoy my weekend. After all, worrying and stressing would not change the outcome, whatever it may be. I have heard about women who have spotting in early pregnancy and have gone on to have healthy pregnancies. I have read that spotting can be completely normal. For me however, it has always been the beginning of a miscarriage. I phoned the early pregnancy unit to tell them about it and was booked in for an emergency scan. We didn't really discuss it any further apart from when Scoop would check in with me and ask how the bleeding was and if it was heavier. There wasn't much else to discuss so we carried on as if everything was okay.

We travelled home to Kent on the Sunday evening and on Monday we arrived at the EPU early ready for the scan. The spotting had turned to bleeding and I was fully prepared to be told that I was miscarrying. Fortunately, it was my favourite nurse doing the scan which made things a little easier. At six weeks pregnant, I had to have a trans-vaginal scan. Just as we had expected, the nurse informed us that there was no sign of a pregnancy in the uterus. This confirmed our seventh pregnancy loss. While we sat in the darkened room which was barely lit by the ultrasound screen Scoop gave me a reassuring squeeze of the hand, but I could see his sadness. There were no tears though, they had already been shed a couple of days prior when the spotting began. We were upset but we had prepared ourselves for this. We knew we were miscarrying again. However, I was not prepared for what came next. Following a scan of the uterus, it is usual practice to check the ovaries and fallopian tubes and it was then that they found the pregnancy. I had what was called a cornual ectopic pregnancy that was found on the left side. It is a rare and dangerous type of ectopic pregnancy that occurs at the junction of the fallopian tube and the uterus. There are different treatment options for this. We could watch and wait to see if it resolved itself, take medications to expel the pregnancy or have the pregnancy surgically removed. However, the treatment option was not my decision this time. Based on the size of the pregnancy and hormone levels in the blood I was left with only one option. I needed to have an operation to remove the Fallopian tube and the affected part of the uterus. This is when the tears came. I went from feeling sad but in control of the situation to feeling completely overwhelmed. I was shocked and shaken; as if our struggles to have a baby were not difficult enough... now this. I just felt like the world was against us. Was this really happening to us? It was a long wait for surgery. I sat all day feeling sorry for myself, for us. We hadn't really told anyone about this pregnancy, I think it's because I had initially felt so positive about it because of the dark line on the pregnancy test.

The problem with not telling anyone that you are pregnant in the first place is that if/when everything goes wrong sharing bad news is much harder than sharing good news. Scoop had to call our family and tell them that we were pregnant but weren't anymore and I required another operation and this time they wouldn't just remove the pregnancy but the tube as well. The operation was done as an emergency (due to the risk of it rupturing) at 10pm that night. I struggled with the recovery. I was transferred from theatre to a general surgical ward where the average age was about 83. I don't cope well with general anaesthetic and I struggle with strong pain relief, it makes me feel really unwell. I spent the night vomiting and crying in pain (I think this was caused by the trapped wind). My little sister sat there with me most of the night and I am very grateful for that, she is such a kind soul. She too is a nurse and that night she really looked after me. She got me pain relief when I needed it, anti-sickness medications as well and she held my hair back while I was vomiting. I felt so unwell that I wasn't able to manage this myself. I have often wondered if the physical recovery of the operations is tougher due to the emotional burden. I have never had an operation that wasn't fertility or gynaecology related so I don't really know. However, I know that my emotions are often all over the place and I am much more sensitive following anaesthesia.

I was discharged home the following evening as I wasn't well enough to leave before that but wasn't keen to stay another night. I walked the familiar walk along the hospital corridor. It was the same corridor that new parents walked to take their tiny babies home in giant car seats. The corridor that was in all those pictures on Facebook to announce that the baby had arrived safely and they were on their way home to start their life together as a family. I wondered if I would ever walk these corridors with Scoop carrying a car seat holding a new baby, our baby. If I did, I would be sure to take a thousand photos. When they discharged me, I was told that due to a reduction in the size of my uterus and the number of previous operations, I would not be able to give birth naturally now. In future pregnancies I would require a planned caesarean section as it was unlikely that my uterus would be able to cope with the force of contractions. My biggest fear was that I would wake up from the anaesthetic with no uterus at all (that had been recorded on the consent form), so in comparison, a c-section didn't seem so bad. It was a bit of a shock because it wasn't mentioned before surgery, but it was absolutely bearable. If I am completely honest, the thought of labour has always absolutely petrified me, as I am sure it does most people. I have always been scared that I would reach a point where it is too much and I cannot push anymore. I've had nightmares about running out of energy or being in too much pain to push anymore and then being shouted at by midwives because the baby is compromised. It was a real fear of mine. I thought of the caesarean section as the easy way out but was pleased that I didn't have to choose to have one because the decision was taken out of my hands.

Following the initial night of feeling terrible in hospital, physically I recovered well at home and I was looked after by my friends and family. Emotionally I expected it to hit me like a ton of bricks at some point but at the time I seemed to be coping well and was quite pragmatic about the whole situation. It's strange, I don't know why but I felt like my grief was more valid this time and because of this I coped rather well, considering. To other people this one seemed more devastating than the other miscarriages or at least that is the reaction I received and everyone was more sympathetic and understanding than previously. It's almost like the grief was justified but in turn this meant that its impact wasn't as huge for me, mentally anyway. I guess it was the trauma of losing a tube and the fertility problems this could cause that made this more significant. Having part of the uterus taken away and the associated risk with carrying any future baby to term, also played on mind. In hindsight it had more of a momentous impact on my fertility and I guess that is why it got the reaction it did. To turn it all on its head, the early miscarriages I had previously were incredibly hard for me to deal with. There was not really anything there for me to grieve for at these times and I think that is why I found them difficult. The only proof that these pregnancies existed was a positive pregnancy test. Everything else there was to mourn for after these losses was created in my head over a few weeks. I imagined what the baby would be like, who they would look like, their name, gender, favourite colour, favourite dinosaur, career, hobbies etc. All of this was created in my imagination. It sort of felt like I was sadder than I should have been and had no real right to feel so devastated, which in turn made me more devastated. It caused a whirlwind of emotions so the ectopic felt like a breeze in comparison. I have no idea if this makes any sense, but it is how I felt.

I had a couple of weeks off work to recover physically, during which time I binged on box sets, ate junk food and chilled with our beloved Cooper.

ABOUT YOU

How would you feel if you were told by a health professional that you couldn't have children? What would you do? Would you look into other ways of becoming a parent or accept childlessness, focusing on other things instead? _____

_____

_____

_____

_____

_____

_____

_____

_____

_____

_____

A TURNING POINT

I counted down the days to the appointment at the miscarriage clinic. We had waited for six months for this appointment. I was so hopeful that this would be the answer for us but at the same time I had my doubts. Scoop and I attended the appointment together. The clinic was running behind schedule, which was apparently normal, so there would be a long wait. We sat in a waiting room full of couples who all looked up when we entered the room. We then did the same whenever a new couple arrived. I guess it's just human nature. I wondered what all these other couples had been through. Were they all here for the same reason or could some of these women already be pregnant? If they were, they weren't showing yet, it would have to be early stages. I was so excited to be called through to see the consultant but equally nervous as I was worried that I would leave disappointed with the outcome like with the previous consultant. It felt like all our hopes and dreams were pinned on the next 20 minutes.

In the room there was the consultant, his registrar and a specialist nurse. They took a very thorough medical history from me. They focused on each individual loss, going into detail about each one and I really felt like they listened to me. I have been looked after by some lovely doctors and nurses who have been very professional, kind and caring however this was the first time that I felt like I was being taken seriously in respect of the recurrent miscarriages. I left the room with a plan and felt positive that we were going to get some answers. I had to have blood tests, many of which I'd had previously, however there were also several autoimmune tests they were doing that I had never had before. The phlebotomist took 15 vials of blood from me and I had to wait for 6 weeks to get these results at my next appointment in the clinic.

I had to consider what would happen if all the tests came back 'normal'. We were pretty certain that we were not prepared to keep trying unless there was a change to our treatment plan. This was our last chance to get some answers or reasons as to why this kept happening to us and hopefully get some help on how to go forward. We couldn't carry on losing more pregnancies, we wouldn't cope with it individually or as a couple. If we were going to be told that it was just bad luck, then this would mean the end of trying for a baby naturally and we would be heading down the adoption route. In fact, I was so tired and fed up of trying to have a baby myself that I was rather eager to get going with adoption.

I just wanted someone (a health professional/specialist in the field) to tell me to give it up already. I wanted to be told that it was never going to happen for us and I felt like I would welcome any advice to move on from TTC. There was something quite satisfying about the feeling of acceptance that our journey was over and I truly felt at peace with this. I knew that I had tried my damndest to have a baby. It had been years of upset, stress and heartache but all options had been explored and enough was enough. I couldn't do it anymore. I was physically, mentally and emotionally exhausted.

When we got the results of the tests we found out that we may actually have an answer and after several years of testing we had hopefully found the reason for our pregnancy losses. After all of these years suspecting that the losses are autoimmune related, it appears I was correct as there were antibodies present in my blood. As strange as it sounds I was over the moon that there was something wrong with me. This diagnosis was also incredibly frustrating as I felt that I could have had these tests done sooner, receiving speedier treatment, probably preventing some of the losses. Anyhow, putting all of that to the back of my mind and focusing on the here and now, I was so pleased that it was something that could be treated simply with tablets. It wasn't just bad luck and it's unlikely that I would have had a successful pregnancy without medical support and medications. Of course, there was still the chance of a 'bad egg' but with the appropriate medications it would mean that a 'good egg' would have as good a chance as anyone else's and the risk of miscarriage would be reduced. I just felt like it was now possible whereas before it seemed absolutely impossible.

I needed to have repeat tests done in three to four months to be sure of the results, before starting the treatment. There was nothing that we could do about this wait, but at least there was now hope. We were told not to TTC for six months. They would do more tests and then I would start treatment and be on the medications for a couple of months before we could TTC again. This in itself was a very strange position for us to be in, particularly after such a long time of doing the opposite. It was so frustrating that we had to wait when we had already waited so long, but I guess it had already been six years. What was another six months?

I endeavoured to develop a positive attitude in the meantime and tried to be thankful for all that I had. I made a conscious effort to enjoy all the good things in my life. As time was ticking on and our chances of having a baby were getting slimmer, it was important that I begin to focus on other things and celebrate my own achievements. Better this than to dwell on what is missing and live a life engulfed in sadness and resentment. It is just not healthy for the mind, body or soul and certainly would not benefit our relationship. Changing my outlook and my focus really helped me. I still had days when I felt sad, after all we had lost seven pregnancies and years down the line I still did not have the one thing I longed for in life. However, I had lots of other wonderful things. I had a kind and loving husband, a roof over my head and I was thankful for going to bed with a full tummy every night. We have always had a large and wonderful support network of family and friends and of course our doting doggy Cooper who we looked forward to coming home to every evening. We worked hard and played hard too. Our jobs are not the most fulfilling, but they afford us the lifestyle we live and neither of us dreads going to work. We would enjoy holidays, weekends away, countryside walks, a few too many take-aways, family gatherings and nights out with friends. We also had lots to look forward to which helped to distract us. I am honoured to be a godmother and blessed to be an aunty. I love being a part of their lives and I look forward to seeing them all develop and grow into lovely little people and I hope to be able to support them and their parents as they navigate the tricky times. I was always waiting to have my own children to be able to enjoy spending time with them, but there was no need to wait, I didn't need to miss out. No-one was stopping me, apart from me.

I had to switch off from baby-making mode and tried to turn my attention to something else. I started exercising more in an attempt to become a healthier and happier version of me and to get myself into the best possible shape for TTC once we were given the go ahead. I played netball already, but I also started running with the dog in the evenings and got back into rowing, all of which kept me pretty busy.

Getting back in the rowing boat reminded me of the summer when Scoop and I first met. It was through mutual friends. Some of the lads he played rugby with had got involved with the rowing club in the summer of 2008. We first met on a night out with rowing friends. It was only a few weeks until we were dating and I have never looked back. I did say at the beginning that I would explain how Scoop acquired his name, it was before we met. He tells me that after a rugby game there would be drinking challenges and one of them involved a Woolworth's pick 'n' mix scoop. It would get shoved into your mouth and then people would pour random booze into it. Apparently, Scoop was quite good at this and it became his tour name. It stuck. We've been through some of the toughest times together and there have been occasions when I was sure that this would break us but we've grown closer and become stronger.

Fast forward 10 years to the summer of 2018 when we waited those few months for more testing. We also bought our first home together in the June of that year, so we spent a lot of time packing up the old house and unpacking the new one. It was a good distraction from the break from TTC. Sometimes we spend too much time and energy focusing on things that we have no control over, so instead we made a conscious effort to keep ourselves busy, sorting out the house and keeping active. We hoped that the months would fly by. Ideally the second lot of tests would confirm the diagnosis, we would then start the treatment and be able to start trying for a baby again at the beginning of 2019. Everything was crossed.

The other thing that helped distract me from the waiting was writing. I cannot stress enough how much it helped me to write down my thoughts, feelings and experiences. I started writing after our sixth loss, in my loneliest times. Writing everything down really did drag me out of a very deep dark hole. To begin with I just wrote down how I felt and what had happened. I set up a blog online but I didn't publish it or show it to anyone to start with. As I wrote more entries in the blog and opened up to a few friends and family about it, I ended up forwarding them the link but with strict instructions that it was for their eyes only. It was following the ectopic pregnancy that I posted it on social media for anyone and everyone to read. I was petrified to do it because I felt ashamed and embarrassed of my inability to carry a baby. I was fed up of feeling inferior to people who could have babies. I knew other people had experienced pregnancy losses too but why was everyone so sheepish and quiet about it. The 'brushing under the carpet' attitude that society has to miscarriage and pregnancy loss definitely contributed to my difficulties in dealing with my grief and it's probably that which spurred me to go public with the blog.

I felt incredibly vulnerable putting myself and our experiences out there for all to read but the outpouring of messages of love and support following this was amazing. I felt like my losses were acknowledged and my grief was valid. So many people reached out to me to tell me of their experiences of miscarriage and infertility. There were people that I know and complete strangers that messaged me about their losses and their fertility problems. For many of them, they had not spoken to anyone about their experiences other than their partner or maybe their best friend or parents. Some people had never told a soul. They too felt embarrassed and inadequate, like their body was useless, it had failed them or they had done something wrong. It was these messages that kept me writing. The more we speak about it, the easier it becomes for others to speak about. In 2018 it really should not have been a taboo subject. It affects so many people. So many! The statistics show that one in four pregnancies end in miscarriage. Tommy's say that 85% of these are first trimester miscarriages (Tommy's, 2018). I have a group of friends that were colleagues and university buddies originally but are wonderful friends now. We go away to Center Parcs most years and it was on our weekend away last year (2019) at Elveden Forrest that we had a discussion about miscarriages. As nurses we tend to be very open and we are used to sharing with each other. Between the six of us we have 13 living children and we have lost 17 pregnancies, at least one each. None of us have escaped miscarriage. Okay so my losses account for many of these, but even so, that is more than one in four.

I have wondered if miscarriages are more common now than before and having done a bit of research it is still unclear. There are a couple of things to consider. The statistics say that numbers of reported miscarriages have increased over the years however it seems that this is likely due to the use of home pregnancy tests (Lang and Nuevo-Chiquero, 2012). Women are now able to confirm their pregnancy very early on and the risk of miscarriage is highest in these very early weeks. If the woman is not aware of her pregnancy then an early miscarriage could go unnoticed and therefore unrecorded. Although it is unreasonable that home pregnancy tests directly affect the risk of miscarriage, the point is that their use could affect the frequency with which women recognise and report them. My mum tells me that she hasn't had any miscarriages, but she had to wait until seven weeks to find out that she was carrying me. So it is very possible that she did have a miscarriage but just wasn't aware of it, after all the majority of my losses were before 7 weeks. Maternal age could also be playing a big part in the rate of miscarriages as the risk increases significantly as we get older. Factors such as the availability of contraception and encouragement to use it as well as the female focus on career progression could all be contributing towards women having babies later in life. This is just food for thought.

After going public with the blog, we were overwhelmed by all the love, support and words of hope and encouragement that we received after being open and honest about our story. However, there were some reactions which were not so positive. Some people distanced themselves from us and in some circles we were left out of things. I guess people were trying to protect us from awkward situations but in doing so it made things even more awkward. I can see now that our friends and family were only ever trying to protect our emotions but at the time it just felt insensitive. I never intended to make people feel like they couldn't talk to us about their children or get excited about their pregnancies. It's just that it was difficult seeing other people in the position that we so desperately wanted to be in, as it highlighted to us what we were missing out on. We were happy for them but also really sad for ourselves. We love children and absolutely adore all the kiddies in our lives. The last thing we wanted was for our struggles to cause any distance between us and our family and friends. Of course it was hard for us, but such is life. People will always have babies and this was our issue to deal with and to get our heads around. We didn't want others to feel burdened by knowing our struggles, we just wanted people to be normal with us. We hoped that they would just bear in mind our struggles and understand that there may be times that we needed to take a step back and withdraw slightly to protect our emotions. Despite this, it felt good to let it all out in the open.

The lines of communication need to be open. Infertility, miscarriage and pregnancy loss are some of the most isolating experiences that people go through. We need to talk to each other, support each other and be a little more understanding.

One day it could happen to you, someone you know or someone you love, and you would not want them to feel so lonely during such tough times. You would want them to feel like they can openly discuss their feelings and grieve if they need to. We need to make it commonplace for these discussions to be had.

ABOUT YOU

You can do this as a one-off activity or try to ask yourself these questions every week or maybe just when you are feeling low. Write down 3 things you...

have accomplished:

are grateful for:

are lucky to have:

appreciate:

really love:

are learning about yourself:

PUTTING FRUSTRATIONS ASIDE

During the six-month break from TTC we waited for our second round of blood tests. We were pleased to know what was wrong and what was causing our losses but had to wait for another set of tests before starting the treatment. Imagine our shock and anxiety when we found out that we were pregnant during this break. We weren't actively TTC because we had been advised not to, so I avoided tracking my cycles and I bought some condoms, which were safely packed in one of the boxes for moving to the new house. We were lucky to be able to take our time with moving, thanks to my dad being our landlord at the old house. We moved all our things ourselves in my car and Scoop's van in the evenings after work over a two-week period. It happened to be the same two weeks of the 2018 heat wave. As you can imagine, sex wasn't at the top of our agenda so it only happened twice that month, but do you think we could find those bloody condoms? Of course not. We should have been more careful really but what were the chances?

It's amazing how much recurrent loss can affect subsequent pregnancies. The usual joy and excitement is not there. It is replaced by stress, worry and a feeling of dread. I am resentful about this. I feel as though I have been cheated out of those happy feels and prevented from enjoying pregnancy. I didn't even phone Scoop to tell him, I just sent him a picture of a positive test.

I was four weeks and six days when I did the test and found out that I was pregnant. This is about a week after I would normally find out. Usually I am tracking my cycles and testing as soon as the tests will pick up a result, normally 10 days post ovulation. My cycles had lengthened over the last couple of months so I hadn't suspected that I might be pregnant until I was at work that Thursday. I had sore boobs and was constantly popping to the loo for a wee throughout the morning. I would usually work through lunch but this particular day I was super hungry, so I popped along to Boots to grab a meal deal. While I was there, I picked up a two-pack of pregnancy tests. I was in a rush so ate my egg mayo and tomato sandwich while walking back to work and then did the test as soon as I got back. It was after this that I texted Scoop. But he wasn't the first person I told. I had confided in one of my colleagues when I saw the specialist the first time in April and she was the first person that I told about my BFP. I guess it was because she was there. I was heading back to my room from having done the test in the toilet and she had her door open and I just blurted it out. I think I was in disbelief. She is a doctor and with a level head she congratulated me but also reminded me that I should call the clinic and let them know as soon as possible.

I called the specialist that afternoon. If there was something wrong with me and I needed medical help to hold onto this pregnancy then I wanted that help as soon as possible. I couldn't deal with another loss. Thankfully, they started me on the treatment straight away. The following day I drove the 90-minute journey each way to collect a very large bag of medication. I was taking nine tablets and two pessaries each day and there were some less than pleasant side effects to begin with, but I would have tried anything if there was a chance of avoiding a miscarriage. This wasn't the treatment that was originally indicated because I hadn't had that second set of blood tests done, so the other medications could not be prescribed. However, this was their standard regime and I was happy to give it a go. Funnily enough it is the exact same treatment that I had asked for a few years ago after my fifth loss, when seeing one of the other specialists; the dismissive one in fact. It turned out that it wasn't 'just bad luck' and despite being 'still young' at the time, having a baby was never going to be successful without this medication. Saying, 'It will happen' was just fobbing me off. If only we could have had the treatment a few years before, it might have saved a fallopian tube, a few friendships and so much heartache.

I've said it before and I will say it again: my advice to anyone TTC and dealing with recurrent pregnancy loss, is to fight for answers! I knew that no amount of 'keep trying' or 'it will happen when you least expect it' would ever result in me having a baby. I knew deep down that there was something else going on. I was patient to begin with and went along with policies and protocols but after a while I knew that it wasn't just bad luck! I did my research, presented the facts to my GP and pushed for a referral and more tests. When that didn't work, I did more research and pushed for more referrals and tests. There were many times when I felt like I was banging my head against a brick wall and wanted to give up. I felt like very few of the many health professionals that we saw were actually on our side or really cared if we had a baby or not but I will be forever grateful to the ones that were. I felt like I was just another patient, a statistic. I fought my own battles and I encourage those going through similar struggles to do the same. Of course it is tough but if the health professionals are not fighting for you then you must find the courage to stand up for yourselves and persevere until you get the answers you need.

I had to put my frustration about all of this aside so we could focus on this pregnancy. There was no point dwelling on the past and being resentful that I couldn't have the tests and treatment earlier, I had them now and for now I was pregnant. I even had a scan picture to prove it, the very first picture of one of my babies, finally! I was still so sure that it would go wrong but to try and muster some positivity we started announcing our pregnancy to close family and friends. We wrote a list of all the people we told so that it would be easy to un-tell everyone if I miscarried again. We received the results of the 12 weeks blood test screening for Downs, Edwards, Patau's syndrome. The screening showed that the foetus was at low risk of having any of these syndromes and I had multiple scans which showed that it was developing normally so far. It was after these results that we shared our news with others. This is what I posted when we announced it on social media.

It has been 5 years, 11 months and 2 days since I had my contraceptive implant removed and we began trying for a baby. In the past 2163 days we have had 5 first trimester miscarriages, an ectopic pregnancy and a partial molar pregnancy. The molar pregnancy involved fortnightly testing by the haemato-oncology unit for 6 months, during which time we were not allowed to TTC (try to conceive). Most recently, in January this year, I had a cornual ectopic pregnancy resulting in the removal of my left fallopian tube and the affected corner of the uterus. So we have had 7 pregnancy losses in total. We have seen 4 different miscarriage specialists at clinics in 4 different hospitals and had multiple investigations. I've endured 3 further gynaecological operations (planned and emergency). Two to remove the 'products of conception' after the pregnancy failed and one resection on my 'heart shaped' womb. I've had countless amounts of blood tests and internal scans and taken a variety of combinations of medications in the form of tablets, injections and pessaries. It has been a long hard journey so far and it is a journey that has changed us both individually and as a couple.

The journey has been devastating and at times it has almost exhausted my emotional reserve. Throughout it all we have tried our best to act normal, to Keep Calm and Carry On, as they say. We no longer get excited about a positive pregnancy test, we are pessimistic and expect the worst to happen and I live in constant fear of others announcing their own joyful news because of the awful feelings of sadness and resentment that this brings. However, some positives have come from our experiences. Most importantly we have become a stronger couple having faced so much loss together. But also, by being open about our experiences we hope to have provided some support for others in similar situations. It was important for me to speak out about our story to make others feel less alone and to help break the silence surrounding recurrent pregnancy loss and miscarriages. It is these other people, those with empty arms, TTC or experiencing loss, that I feel like I must apologise to for what is coming next.

I feel some guilt about doing this because I know how much it would have upset me but equally I wanted to share our story to give others some hope. I know that it's hard to remain hopeful when all you have experienced is loss but what kept me going was hearing positive stories from others who had also navigated this journey of recurrent loss. So this is for those women.

I believe it is about time we had some luck and happiness. That is not to say that all those currently struggling don't deserve this too. You know who you are. You deserve this! It's not fair, it sucks and I'm truly so sorry you are in this bloody awful club that no one wants to be a part of.

So anyway, here goes... It fills me with great joy and some trepidation to announce that we are expecting our rainbow baby in March. Today *marks 14 weeks into the pregnancy. So hopefully, thanks to a new treatment plan, we will get to meet this little one next year.*

Our family and close friends have known about this for a while now. We have needed their support. It has been an anxious, stressful and worrying time. We have never had an embryo that survived past 8 weeks before, let alone graduate to an actual foetus. I never thought I would ever reach the second trimester, yet here we are! I was scanned 6 times before my 12 week dating scan, mostly for reassurance purposes but also due to some bleeding and other concerning symptoms. I guess lots of people have these symptoms and from speaking to others I realise that even those who have not experienced a single loss, will have similar anxieties. I think mine are just exacerbated by my experiences. With every scan I had, I was expecting bad news. 'Scanxiety' is a real thing. I expected to hear those words that we have heard so many times before... 'I'm sorry, there is no heartbeat'.

In fact at 12 weeks I had a big bleed and was so sure that it was all over. We sat in the waiting room of the EPU and Smooth FM radio was on in the background. The Foreigner song 'I want to know what love is' came on...

'In my life there's been heartache and pain, I don't know if I can face it again...'

I sobbed. I was so sure of the news I would be getting. I was already thinking about how we would tell everyone we had miscarried again and I was considering whether I would have medical management or surgery to remove the failed pregnancy. I was so unbelievably shocked at what I saw on the ultrasound screen. There was a beating heart and the arms and the legs were kicking and waving. I honestly could not believe it. You can imagine our relief!

Anyway, so far so good. I still can't shake the anxiety, however it is slowly being taken over by some excitement and an awful lot of hope, which was previously in very short supply. I never thought I would enjoy pregnancy because of all that has happened to us and for the most part I don't, but it's growing on me. The whole experience of pregnancy is tainted by what has happened to us in the past but I am learning to be positive and even made my first baby purchase at the weekend (a very cute hungry caterpillar outfit). It could all go horribly wrong tomorrow but the chances of something bad happening are getting slimmer and each day I am one step closer. Today I am pregnant and I will celebrate that with a glass of chocolate milk. Cheers!

Clicking the button to post this announcement on Facebook and Instagram was absolutely petrifying but within minutes we had messages of congratulations, love and support flooding in.

ABOUT YOU

How would you prefer to be told/find out about someone's pregnancy announcement? It might depend who it is. If you can identify what will upset you or a way that will make it less triggering for you then tell people. Hopefully they will respect your honesty and honour the request.

_____

_____

_____

_____

_____

_____

_____

_____

_____

_____

COPING WITH PREGNANCY AFTER LOSS

It wasn't how I had always imagined announcing our pregnancy but then I am well aware that things don't always work out as you imagine them to. The third time we got pregnant, all those years before, I had planned to announce in a different way. I was due to be reaching 12 weeks around the time of Halloween. After two scans where we saw the heart beating we had let ourselves get excited and got carried away about how we would tell everyone that we were finally expecting. I've never thought I would be one to make an extravagant announcement but having had two early pregnancy losses prior to this I felt like it was deserved and justified. So, with that in mind I went about buying pumpkins and some booties in preparation for our announcement picture. We had a big pumpkin to signify Daddy, a slightly smaller one to signify me and a tiny one to signify the little baby that I was carrying. We put our shoes and the booties next to the appropriate pumpkins and took lots of pictures. We had planned to wait until after our dating scan to announce on social media, but the pictures were ready so that we could post them straight away. I was so excited to tell the world about our 'third time lucky' baby. Obviously we never got to share these pictures as this was the molar pregnancy and in my anger and grief I deleted them, along with every picture that I had taken of the hundreds of positive pregnancy tests. I never prepared any other pictures for announcements of subsequent pregnancies either. I feel like I have been cheated out of being able to prepare an announcement picture. Not just that but I feel like there are several things that I can't/won't do now, having gone through what we have. There are two reasons for this. The first reason is protecting the feelings of other people and the second reason is superstition. I feel like I would have been jinxing myself, tempting fate and ultimately making the bad news so much worse after attempting to be positive and hopeful about it. It's like a self-preservation mode; don't get attached and then it won't hurt as much when you lose it; don't acknowledge it as being real or exciting and it won't be as devastating when you receive that bad news. I hate that I thought like this. I hate that recurrent pregnancy loss made me like this.

One of the other things that I wouldn't do was have a baby shower. Having attended various baby showers in the past there came a point when I had to stop going to them because it was making me depressed and anxious. I feel incredibly guilty about not attending some of my closest friend's baby showers and family members for that matter, but again this was self-preservation. Now this might come across as controversial, but I think baby showers are silly anyway. I have several issues with them. Firstly, what if the baby does not arrive safely? Anything can happen in those late stages of pregnancy and it does.

Secondly, the baby shower is an American tradition whereby you shower the mum-to-be in gifts prior to the baby's arrival. Well whatever happened to visiting with a gift once the baby had arrived safely? Or are we meant to do both now? At the baby showers I have been to everyone sits around drinking prosecco and watches the mum-to-be open all her gifts in front of everyone. I find this rather cringey and incredibly showy. Then you play a game where you have to guess if the picture is of a woman who is in labour or in a porn movie. The event finishes off with cakes or if you are really lucky there are some melted chocolate 'poos' squished up inside nappies and you have to guess the chocolate bar. Now don't get me wrong, I do like cake but the rest of it I feel is just very pretentious and it's not my kind of thing.

Now I have actually considered if my reasons for disliking baby showers are more to do with my own issues of bitterness, jealousy and resentment. I don't know the answer to this. I will never know because I cannot erase my experiences. However, when I made my decision not to have a baby shower it was primarily due to protecting the feelings of others who I know are battling with pregnancy loss and infertility themselves. Knowing how it makes me feel to get an invite to one, I knew how it would make others feel and for the sake of a few generic presents I did not want to put anyone else through that. When I caught wind of a surprise baby shower being organised for me, I put a stop to it straight away. At the time I couldn't think of anything worse.

I wouldn't hold it against anyone who has a baby shower, after all rarely does anyone organise their own 'buy me presents for my baby' party, it is usually organised on their behalf and I get it, it's exciting. You might think that being in our situation would make it even more exciting and it would be an extra special situation. I just think that maybe a nice afternoon tea or meal with friends/family as a 'final hoorah' before baby comes is more reasonable. Then they can all come and visit you for cuddles when the baby is actually here. I planned a 'last supper' with a handful of my local friends as it would be the last time I would be able to do that for some time as I was planning on breast feeding. We just went for an all-you can-eat Chinese meal and I insisted on no presents although I think a couple of the girls broke the rules but I left them in the car and opened them at home with Scoop.

My anxiety was sky high during this meal as it had been for the whole pregnancy in fact. This anxiety was for a good reason and I will discuss this shortly when I tell you what happened the following day. The trouble is that when the only experiences you have of pregnancy involve loss, you think and hope that the next pregnancy will help resolve the feelings of fear, bitterness and sadness. However, in reality, those feelings are still bubbling away and occasionally they rise to the surface. Even if everything is going to plan and you have been given no cause for concern, you still doubt that you will get the desired outcome. Pregnancy after loss is so bittersweet. Feelings of hope and optimism are tainted by those of anxiety and uncertainty. You try to let yourself get excited but anything can trigger the negative thoughts that bring you crashing back down to the reality of 'this baby might not make it' and 'why would it work this time when it hasn't so many times before?'

Over the years, I doubted if my body was actually capable of making and carrying a baby. After all, my track record was pretty bad. In the early stages of this pregnancy the only thing that kept me sane was knowing that I was finally on tablets that should stop my body rejecting this baby that I so desperately wanted. I had to try to remain positive and with every milestone we reached, I reminded myself that the tablets were doing their job. Once I reached the second trimester I knew that we had passed the point of our previous losses and therefore this pregnancy was unlikely to end for the same reasons as before. The third trimester brought with it the reassurance that if the baby was to come from then on, there was an increasing likelihood that it would survive so every extra day of pregnancy was a bonus. However, I still doubted if it would actually result in bringing our baby home.

There were a few other things that helped me with my anxiety during this pregnancy which I will share in the hope that they may help someone else.

Lots of scans and appointments

I was monitored closely by the early pregnancy unit for the first 12 weeks and they were very supportive. I also had some private scans that we paid for or were gifted by friends that understood our anxieties. In total, I had 14 scans and attended the foetal assessment unit several times with reduced movements of the baby. I had an anterior placenta (at the front) so I felt very few movements anyway but with my history of recurrent pregnancy loss the staff were always happy to help and understanding about having extra checks to confirm everything was okay and ease my anxieties. I had a couple of appointments with the obstetric team to discuss the planned caesarean and I was discharged from the reproductive immunologist at 16 weeks. Other than that input, I was treated as a normal pregnancy and it was progressing as it should. It was the reduced movements that resulted in the increased input towards the end of the pregnancy. Being at the hospital and having lots of input really helped me. Just to know that the baby was okay (especially with feeling very few movements) was very reassuring.

Taking it one day at a time

I would count down the days from one scan or appointment to the next. I looked forward to seeing the midwife so that I could hear the heartbeat on the Doppler machine. We followed the baby's development on some apps on my phone and looked forward to

Wednesdays so that we could see what fruit or vegetable our baby was a similar size too. I had to take it day by day and that is the only way I managed to stay sane throughout. I tried to celebrate small milestones, even when I had my doubts and felt fearful about what was to come. With time and with each milestone, it became more real and the anxiety eased a little. I'll never forget the day I was given my maternity notes, that was a first for us and being able to send our scan picture to people was also pretty special as we had never got to do this before. Celebrate the small victories and acknowledge all the milestones.

Sharing my anxieties

I was quite open about my anxiety and I shared my thoughts and worries with my husband, friends and family. But when everyone around you is so excited and optimistic, it can be difficult to express your true feelings without feeling like you are being pessimistic and constantly bringing down the mood. Towards the end of my pregnancy I found myself just agreeing with people when they would ask me about how excited I was feeling. This appeared to be the preferred response as opposed to my real answer of something along the lines of 'anything could happen, I won't believe it until the baby is safely in my arms'. I found it really helpful to talk about my fears and doubts with other ladies (and a few men) who had been through similar experiences and I received great support from some truly wonderful people from baby/rainbow/miscarriage groups on social media. Support from others can just feel empty if they've not been through it themselves. The baby loss and miscarriage communities online are just fantastic. It is a secret club, a club that no-one wants to be a part of, but it is a club that you need your membership to if you find yourself experiencing pregnancy loss. There is something truly empowering about talking to people who just get it. They understand your darkest thoughts, they've had them too. I hope you don't have to join this club, but if you do, or you know anyone who does, don't be scared to reach out.

Self-care

Yes, I am jumping on this bandwagon! The concept is not new but the importance of it appears to be. Thank goodness, it's almost as if we now have permission to look after ourselves; body and mind. I tried not to put too much pressure on myself to feel attached or enjoy the pregnancy. That was always going to be a battle and I couldn't help but remain slightly distant from this thing that I had always dreamed of which was growing inside me. I did however try to focus on making the pregnancy a healthy one. This is where the self-care comes in. I let my attention drift from work somewhat and my priorities were rest, sleep and nutrition. I was too scared to carry on with sport and exercise when I found out I was pregnant. I was playing netball, running and had taken up rowing again when I fell pregnant this time however my paranoia about losing the baby got the better of me so dog walking was my only real regular physical activity, but it was better than nothing I guess. As for nutrition, I tried my best to eat healthily and eat foods that were high in iron however my cravings generally took over, but I tried not to feel too guilty about this. The first trimester craving was stodgy foods like beans, southern fried chicken and jacket potatoes with cheese of course! I could have coped with that meal every night. The second trimester was all about fresh orange juice and the third was Belgian buns (however I'm not sure if the latter was an actual craving or a simple desire).

I also tried some mindfulness apps at the beginning of the pregnancy which weren't particularly useful but kept my mind occupied for a while. Anything that helped fill time was a winner, including box sets. I also wrote in a diary every day and found writing in general very helpful. In the latter stages of pregnancy, I had a proper pregnancy massage which was absolutely wonderful and really helped with the swelling in my legs and feet.

Towards the end of the pregnancy we were given lots of things for the baby, from some very kind and generous friends. It was coming up to Christmas so I guess everyone was eager to clear some space at their houses, but I wasn't ready for it to be filling space at ours. As Scoop brought all the things into the house I just sobbed. I wasn't prepared for these feelings. At first I didn't know why I was crying but I soon realised that the tears came because I couldn't imagine us ever having a baby and didn't imagine ever being able to use any of the lovely things and this is what made me desperately sad. It was for this reason that we were a bit slow at getting things ready for the baby. We left most things until the very last minute and there were some things that were not done at all. We didn't decorate the nursery and we bought very few baby clothes and other essentials. I left the packing of my hospital bag until the weekend before the planned caesarean. The beauty of having the date planned in advance is you can count down the days and you know exactly how long you have to get organised. I guess most couples usually savour such tasks but for us they were just too difficult, so we put them off.

The latter stages of pregnancy were really tough, both physically and mentally. I can honestly say that although the anxiety in pregnancy eased with time, I really did not enjoy pregnancy one little bit. I was not able to shake the significant lack of faith in my body's ability to do what it was meant to. Pregnancy was not the joyous experience that I had always dreamed of but that was no real surprise. After all we'd been through I fully expected the experience to be tainted.

I take my hat off to those that manage being heavily pregnant during the summer months as I struggled with our mini February 'heat wave'! I have no idea how I would do it while looking after a toddler or having a physically demanding job. It was really tough, even without any morning sickness (thanks to the steroids). But I won't bore you with all my symptoms and struggles. The purpose of this is not to seek sympathy for my struggles in pregnancy but to explain why I found it tough and why I moaned a lot.

At the beginning of this pregnancy I felt terribly guilty when complaining and I tried to focus on how lucky I was to finally be getting what I had wished for. In the past I always got really annoyed with people complaining about pregnancy. It would drive me crazy to hear people moaning when all I wanted was the chance to hold on to my own pregnancy for more than a couple of months. I thought it was ungrateful and selfish of them. I remember thinking that I would have loved to have had the opportunity to complain about the symptoms caused by a baby growing inside of me.

Now that I've been in that position myself, I get it. It's tough! I'm sorry for being so judgmental. I have a friend who was pregnant at the same time as me, her with her third. She was so happy that I was moaning about my pregnancy symptoms because it meant that she could moan too. Bless her, in her previous two pregnancies she never said a negative word in front of me as she knew how much it would sting to hear it. I was not so good at keeping my complaints to myself. Why? Because it's bloody hard work. People ask you all the time how you are feeling so I think it is okay to answer truthfully and verbalise your struggles to them. If they don't want this answer, they shouldn't ask. However, I really do appreciate how lucky I am to have had the opportunity to moan about these things. I think it is possible to be happy, excited and honoured to be pregnant but still find it difficult at the same time.

I still have awful guilt about my pregnancy complaints because I know how so many would give anything to have been in my shoes. I remain very conscious of other people's feelings as I have been there and fully understand how difficult it is to hear someone moaning about something that you are desperate to experience yourself. Although I didn't enjoy the experience, I'm still grateful for it as it's the reward at the end that makes it all worthwhile.

ABOUT YOU

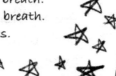

Mindfulness.
Why don't you try this body scan :
This body scan can be performed while sitting. Look on the mindful.org
website to find the audio of this body scan, or you could record yourself
saying these words and play it back.

Begin by bringing your attention into your body.
You can close your eyes if that's comfortable for you.
You can notice your body seated wherever you're seated,
feeling the weight of your body on the chair, on the floor.
Take a few deep breaths.
And as you take a deep breath, bring in more oxygen
enlivening the body. And as you exhale, have a sense of
relaxing more deeply.
You can notice your feet on the floor, notice the sensations of
your feet touching the floor. The weight and pressure,
vibration, heat.
You can notice your legs against the chair, pressure, pulsing,
heaviness, lightness.
Notice your back against the chair.
Bring your attention into your stomach area. If your
stomach is tense or tight, let it soften. Take a breath.
Notice your hands. Are your hands tense or tight. See if you
can allow them to soften.
Notice your arms. Feel any sensation in your arms. Let your
shoulders be soft.
Notice your neck and throat. Let them be soft. Relax.
Soften your jaw. Let your face and facial muscles be soft.
Then notice your whole-body present. Take one more breath.
Be aware of your whole body as best you can. Take a breath.
And then when you're ready, you can open your eyes.

This is a short body scan. There are longer ones online –
just search for mindfulness body scan.

IF IN DOUBT, GET CHECKED OUT

I said I would come back to the all-you-can-eat Chinese meal. It had been arranged for a couple of weeks so despite feeling pretty crappy I forced myself to go. I really had to stop myself from cancelling at the last minute. I've already mentioned that I felt very few movements of the baby due to the anterior placenta and this particular Thursday was no different. I had been out that day and felt a faint flutter at lunchtime but hadn't felt anything else since then. My logic was that if I went to the Chinese meal, all the sugar from the sweet and sour sauce and some cold fizzy coke might get the baby moving. So, I forced myself out of the house to see my friends. I struggled to manage the short walk from the car park to the restaurant. My feet and legs were terribly swollen and I was very short of breath. I had a wet cough and just felt very congested, I had done for several weeks already. I felt no movements for the duration of the meal but thought that maybe it was because I was sat up, chatting and moving around a lot (restless legs meant that I couldn't sit still for long at all in the third trimester). I thought that I was sure to feel something when I was lying down in bed. We didn't stay late and I went to bed as soon as I got home. I still didn't feel any movements. They advise you to attend the hospital if the pattern of the movements change but I never really felt anything so it was hard to tell when to seek help. I'd been at the hospital the day before and baby was fine then, so I was not too concerned.

I usually felt faint movements first thing in the morning but not this day. It was Friday morning, the day after the Chinese meal and I hadn't felt any movements since lunchtime the day before. I was booked in for a planned caesarean section the following Tuesday, only four days away. However, when I woke up in the morning and expressed my concerns to Scoop, I quickly talked myself into going to get checked out. After all I was on maternity leave (only the third day of it mind you) so other than packing my hospital bag and organising baby's wardrobe I had nothing else to do. I kissed Scoop goodbye while he was getting ready for work and I jumped in the car and called the hospital on my way as previously advised.

I arrived at the foetal assessment unit at about 6am and the midwife hooked me up to the CTG (cardiotocography) monitor. I had been through this several times, so I knew the drill by now. I could see the baby's heartbeat on the monitor and I recognised the periods of rapid heartbeat as the baby moving around. The only trouble (the same trouble I had experienced throughout the pregnancy) was that I couldn't feel these movements. On my previous visits to the assessment unit, I had stayed on the monitor for about 30 minutes and providing all was well and they saw enough evidence of movement I was discharged with the advice to contact them again if I had any concerns. However, this time was a bit different. The midwife who was taking care of me had been to see one of the doctors to show them the trace from the monitor. They also read my notes and due to the increased frequency of my visits to the unit in recent weeks, they wanted me to have a quick scan to check that the blood flow through the placenta and to the baby's brain. The midwife reassured me that it was just a formality and they were pretty sure that all would be fine and I would be on my way home soon to get organised for the arrival of the baby on Tuesday.

I headed to the cafe for a decaf coffee and breakfast bap while I waited for the scanning department to open. I hoped that I would be able to get my scan early as I was meeting friends at lunchtime. I had not for a single second considered that I would not be going home to sleep in my own bed that night. However, that is exactly what happened. The scan showed that the amount of fluid around the baby was reduced and then I was told that the blood flow to the baby's brain was not compromised but this was promptly followed by '...yet'. The blood flow in the placenta was not as it should be and could potentially cause further problems. Scoop was at work, but my mum arrived while we waited for a plan from the doctor. The results of the scan were reviewed by the consultant and it was decided that waiting another four days would not be wise. I was to be admitted to the ward for monitoring and was put on the list for an emergency c-section. I was in shock.

This really demonstrates the importance of monitoring the baby's movements and getting checked out if you are worried. The Kicks Count Campaign is doing great work at spreading the message and highlighting the importance of foetal movements. I'll add their website in the support section at the end.

Believe it or not, I hadn't really thought too much about actually having this baby, I truly never really believed we would get to meet it. As my mum and I were ushered through to the ward I had a real mix of emotions and I'm sure my mum did too; she's been on this journey with me from the very beginning. I cancelled my lunch plans with friends and I was anxious and excited when I phoned Scoop at work to tell him the news. When he arrived on the ward there was still a chance that our baby could be arriving that same day however the longer time went on it seemed more likely that it would be a Saturday baby. It didn't really matter to me what day the baby was born as long as it was healthy. However, when we booked in for the planned c-section, I was able to choose the date. I was persuaded by the midwife to choose Tuesday the 12th instead of Wednesday the 13th which would have been exactly 38 weeks gestation. It all seemed so irrelevant now.

Scoop had some help to pack me a hospital bag and have a quick tidy at home while my sister-in-law and Lil-the-lodger organised the baby clothes which I still hadn't got round to even looking at, let alone sorting out. Scoop could have stayed at the hospital with me that night but we knew that he would need his sleep for the next day, so he headed home to get some rest. That night was so surreal, I was incredibly uncomfortable in fact I had been for several weeks by this point, it was the back and hips that were painful. That night I was up and down to the toilet constantly and just couldn't settle. I petrified, overwhelmed and ever so excited too. I think I slept about three hours in total. This reminds me that whenever I mentioned to people about the lack of sleep during pregnancy, they would always say, "You'd better get used to it." I think that it's really unfair that you are prepared for sleep deprivation by more sleep deprivation; surely Mother Nature should let you sleep well in preparation.

The next morning, Saturday 9th March, Scoop arrived early at the hospital as did my mum and sister. We were still unsure of the time for the caesarean section, all I knew was that we were last on the list due to it being less urgent than the other ladies and I was totally fine with that. I was ready for when they would call for me, wearing my stockings and theatre gown. The last time I had been prepared for an operation like this was when I had the ectopic. Inside I was hoping and praying that this time we got to take a baby home. I was a ball of nerves and felt really shivery, even though I was not cold. When they came to say that they were ready for us I just burst into tears. Big ugly tears. Shit! This was it, I was about to meet my baby. The adrenalin rushed through my veins and all I could focus on was that I hadn't felt any movements for almost two days, and although the monitor had shown that all was okay, I doubted if the baby was even still alive. Having seen several caesarean sections while training to be a nurse, I knew that there was every possibility that our baby would need some help with breathing and we might not get to hold it straight away. I have no idea what route of birth is easiest, but I now know that the 'through the sunroof' method is by no means easy. Don't worry, I will spare you all the gory details but I will say that I struggled, big time. Like most women who have a natural birth, following all the drama I swore that I would never do that ever again and I was deadly serious about this.

What I will say is that it was all worth it, for that Lion King moment; that moment when they lifted our screaming baby up over the surgical drapes, like when Rafiki lifted Simba up on Pride Rock for all of the Serengeti to see. I couldn't see if it was a boy or a girl because the down-belows were so swollen. Scoop and I sobbed our little hearts out at the sight of our alive baby. I have never felt so happy and relieved in all my life. We cried so much at first that we couldn't talk to be able to clarify the gender. We had decided to leave the gender as a surprise on the day because we didn't really mind either way. Due to us having a planned caesarean (or so we thought) we would know the date of birth in advance and we knew that if we had known the gender then we would also have a name planned. After all we had been through, we just wanted something to be a surprise. Now although we didn't really mind about the gender, the discussions about names were causing difficulties. Our boy's name was agreed on but we just could not settle on a girl's name. We both had very strong opinions, and those opinions were not the same. While lying on the operating table I had a bit of a freak out while having my tummy cut open. It was at this point that Scoop finally conceded that if it was a girl then I could choose the name considering all that my body was being put through. She would be a Florence. Nevertheless, the baby was a boy and he was placed on my chest while the surgeons went about 'tidying up' my abdomen. It was six minutes from the moment of the first incision to the baby being born but it took an awful lot longer to sew me back up again. This was due to something about trying to fit my bowels back in. I didn't ask any more details about this. Having our very own baby wriggling around on my chest was incredibly overwhelming and Scoop couldn't wait to tell the world. He was already messaging people while I was still being operated on. In fact, the whole of the Rugby WhatsApp group knew before anyone else because it was close to kick off and Scoop thought that our good news would pep them all up a bit. My mum and sister had been waiting right outside the doors to the delivery suite and they were joined by Scoop's mum and sister too.

It took some time for us to get to the ward but in the meantime, in the recovery room, our mums were allowed to come and see us and meet our little miracle.

Our rainbow baby Albert Charles Lambourne Buckingham was born on 9th March 2019 at 12:47, weighing 5lb 15oz.

It was six and a half years since we started trying for a baby and at times I never thought it would actually happen, yet here he was. What a journey! Miscarriage was tough, recurrent pregnancy loss was torture and pregnancy after loss was horrendous. I'm a different person because of the journey.

I knew it wouldn't sink in until he was actually here and safely in our arms. I just wanted to kiss and cuddle him all day and night. Everyone wanted to meet him and we wanted to show him off to the world. People kept asking me if it felt strange. It didn't. It felt just right.

ABOUT YOU

How did you/would you like to celebrate your
pregnancy?
Would you have a baby shower? Gender reveal?
When and how did you/would you announce the
pregnancy and birth?

_____
_____
_____
_____
_____
_____
_____
_____
_____
_____
_____

MOTHERHOOD AFTER LOSS

Well that's it really, that's our story. That's how we got to the point of having an actual alive baby. From the moment that Bertie was placed on my chest I felt different. I felt like I had a purpose and everything was good again, just as it was meant to be. This was the feeling I had longed for. I hadn't really thought very much about bringing this baby home, caring for it or being its mum, which must sound strange when it was all I had ever dreamed of. Although being a mum was all I had thought about for over six years, I hadn't believed that I would actually get the chance to be one. Even though I hoped everything would be okay, I truly believed it wouldn't be. I didn't allow myself to really think about what happened afterwards, the focus was always on just growing and birthing a healthy baby.

I had such low expectations of motherhood and of myself and my baby. I expected it to be too difficult for me, too tiring and too stressful. I imagined the baby would just cry all the time and

Scoop and I would argue non-stop. I am not sure if it was the long enduring journey to get him or just that he was a very good baby, but nothing really phased me and I treasured every moment of that fourth trimester. I'm not saying it was easy, not at all, it's the hardest thing I've ever had to do but also the best, by far. I'd let myself imagine that it would be a shit show and it wasn't, it was actually quite lovely.

In the process of writing this book, there has been one loss I have struggled with writing about in particular. In 2015, our family suffered a devastating blow when we lost my lovely cousin Charlie. It is hard to put into words what Charlie meant to me, but I want to talk about her here, partly because she was so important and special to me but also because her journey with pregnancy and motherhood is relevant to my own, and it had an impact on what I'll share with you next.

One of my biggest fears was having post-natal mental health problems. Thankfully I have never really struggled too much with my mental health but I know so many people do and I was petrified that I would become one of them. I worried that after all the heartache and pain we had gone through to get a baby, that I wouldn't bond properly or would find the pressure all too much. Almost as if I longed for it so much that I would be disappointed when it actually happened. It was a niggling concern of mine which I felt that I needed to be quite open about so that those around me were ready to see the signs, even if I couldn't.

Charlie and I were very close. I have lots of lovely cousins, but I was closest to Charlie. We were each other's favourite. Although she lived in the West Country and we grew up in Kent, we would spend a lot of the school holidays together either here in Gravesend or there in Somerset and I always looked forward to seeing her. We had great fun at family weddings and holidays in Cornwall. As we got older, we developed a friendship outside of family gatherings. She was a couple of years older than me but she studied medicine for 6 years, so our time at university overlapped and we ended up being at university in London at the same time. We visited each other every few months and spoke and wrote often. That sounds pretty old school doesn't it? But Charlie was very thoughtful, she would send letters and cards often. I, on the other hand, was not the best at reciprocating this but this didn't deter her from continuing to write. When we finished university and moved back home we would make the four-hour journey for weekend visits several times a year and we talked often, every couple of weeks in fact, more so after I returned to university a few years later to do my nurse training. We both worked shifts in hospitals but always found time for a catch up and she was really supportive of me when I experienced my earlier miscarriages. She was one of my go-to people for advice and support. It was my molar pregnancy in 2014 that coincided with her pregnancy. We would have been due only a few weeks apart, but I didn't know about her pregnancy until after mine had ended. She was almost apologetic when she told me about her pregnancy. I struggled with this news because at the time our loss was still very raw. More importantly, there is no one that I would have loved to have been pregnant at the same time as more than her. I wanted our babies to grow up together and to be as close as we were and I felt like I was grieving for the loss of this opportunity. It stirred up a lot of emotion and if I am completely honest, I harboured some resentment about it happening so easily for them and so soon after they started trying.

I distanced myself from her during the pregnancy because I just couldn't face everything. I didn't visit her once while she was pregnant which was easy to get away with because we lived so far from each other and both had busy lives. We were still in contact regularly, but it was more via text than calls. I hated that I was like this, but I was just so low. It was that all important self-preservation. Fast forward to June when she had the baby, I was so excited. Like I have mentioned previously, the bitterness and resentment goes for me when the lovely little bundle arrives. We spoke a few times in the early weeks and I had regular photo updates of her little girl. I was trying to work out a time when we could go to visit and meet the baby. I called her one Saturday but she didn't answer. She messaged me back later saying that she was busy, they were away for the weekend, so she was going to call me back next week. The previous week she had done the same but not returned my call. I didn't think much of it and just assumed she was busy with her new baby. In hindsight I should have seen these signs.

Our worlds came crashing down the following Tuesday (just three days after she had text me) when we were told the news that Charlie had died. I was at work on the ward and was shocked to see my brother and sister-in-law (pregnant at the time) strolling up the corridor. I was doing the medication round at the time and seeing them was initially a nice surprise but then I worried that something was wrong with their baby. What else would they be doing at the hospital? The closer they got the easier it was to see that everything was not okay. They confirmed that their baby was fine but they needed to speak to me about something else. They told me I needed to go with them. I needed to leave work and go to my mum's house. I was frozen in that spot where I was standing. I knew it was something bad but I had no idea what. Was it Mum? Nan? What had happened? I couldn't move. I made them tell me. I was not expecting them to tell me that. 'My Charlie' I wailed. 'Not my Charlie!' My legs felt like jelly and I just sobbed.

It seemed that she had been struggling with her mental health so much that it led her to end her own life. The coroner's conclusion was that her death was a result of suicide and it was presumed that she had been battling postpartum psychosis (also known as puerperal psychosis, PPP). PPP is a rare but serious mental health problem affecting women in the first few weeks/months of motherhood. It is different to post-natal depression in that with PPP there is a significant loss of touch with reality where the woman may hold false beliefs that their life or that of the baby is in danger. It is treated as a medical emergency and can get worse very quickly without any treatment. The symptoms can be difficult to differentiate from the usual behaviours demonstrated during the newborn baby days. The trouble is that those with PPP may not be able to spot the signs themselves because of the effects of the illness itself. The NHS website lists the symptoms as:

- Behaving out of character
- Feeling confused
- Restlessness
- Feeling confused or fearful
- Loss of inhibitions
- Low mood
- Manic mood
- Delusions
- Hallucinations

In the UK help can be sought via the GP, 111, 999, A&E or crisis team. I think it is important for everyone who is around women in those first few months of motherhood to be aware of the symptoms. It might just save someone's life.

Charlie's baby girl was just nine weeks old when she died. It shook our family to the core. I had no idea that anything was wrong, no-one really did. I mean most new mums are exhausted, emotional and it can take a long while for them to get back to their old self, if they ever do at all. I still can't get my head round it, I don't think I ever will. We will never really know what was going through her mind at that time and I will always carry the guilt that maybe if I had not distanced myself then things would have been different. Of course, I know that is unlikely, but I can't help but think like this. Not a single day has passed that I have not thought of her. I miss her terribly, we all do.

I was probably quite ignorant of post-natal mental health problems prior to this but during my own pregnancy it was at the forefront of my mind and it absolutely petrified me. However, I was one of the lucky ones for whom motherhood felt so natural. Bertie was an easy baby and Scoop was wonderful in his new role as a daddy. I was pleasantly surprised at how well Scoop looked after not only Bertie but also me during my recovery from the c-section. We were discharged from the hospital on the Sunday lunchtime. We walked down that all too familiar corridor but this time we were carrying our very own car seat with our very own baby in it. Although we forgot to take the all-important 'car seat in the corridor' picture, all of a sudden that was no longer important. Like a few other things that I had previously placed some importance on, they now seemed insignificant and all that mattered was just having him here, alive.

We made it home within 24 hours of Bertie being born. That drive home was so scary which is strange because I have never experienced Scoop driving that carefully before. I sat in the front of the car so couldn't see him in his rear facing car seat as we hadn't fitted the mirror yet what with him catching us off guard. I was petrified that he would stop breathing and we would not notice because we couldn't see him. My anxiety was sky high at this point but when we arrived home I felt much more at ease. We had lots of visitors, even on the day we arrived home. Lots of people had advised me that we probably wouldn't want visitors for the first couple of weeks and that we should not be shy about saying so but we did want to see people. When people told me this, I remember thinking there was no way we would want to turn people away and I was right. We wanted people to meet Bertie, we were so proud and wanted to show him off to everyone. In fact, I think we probably had in excess of 50 people visit our house in that first two weeks. Scoop was off work, so we were all together. I loved this time in the new-born bubble and it was nice to share it with so many people. We even went to a friend's wedding when he was three weeks old. Of course, there wasn't a great deal of sleep during those early weeks and it took me a little while to get the hang of breast feeding but it was perfect.

Once Scoop went back to work the visitors continued to flow and I started getting out a bit more. Taking Cooper for a walk got me out every day, even if it was just for a short while. I really embraced the fourth trimester, it was all about coffee, cake, naps and cuddles. I would sit and sing 'You are my sunshine' to Bertie while I was feeding him and some days I just sobbed. I was just overwhelmed with how much I loved him and I worried about losing him. Bertie spent a lot of time in the sling carrier and I loved having him close to me. It made me so sad that I had been missing out on this for so many years, but this made Bertie seem even more precious. I made a conscious decision to stop dwelling on the losses and to instead count my blessings. It warmed my heart the day I put him in that 'very hungry caterpillar' baby grow that I had bought him all those months ago, that was the moment that I felt we had succeeded and all would be well.

I felt a bit of pressure to be happy and enjoy every minute of motherhood. I promised myself that I would not moan about a thing. I struggled with pregnancy and moaned about it a lot but I was adamant that once the baby was here that I would not complain at all. I wasn't going to moan about the tiredness, sore boobs or 'poonamis'; I was full of good intentions, I promise. What I hadn't considered was that you (a) don't deal with sleep deprivation better because you've had a miscarriage, (b) mastitis is horrendous despite having lost multiple pregnancies, (c) even if it is a longed for rainbow baby, when they are rolling around in their runny poo while you are changing their nappy it is incredibly fucking irritating. I guess what I mean is that I don't think we are supposed to be attentive during every waking moment and watch with admiration while they sleep. I don't think we are meant to grin and bear the tough moments, just because it was a struggle to have a baby. Getting impatient, snappy, frustrated and annoyed made me feel terribly guilty but it shouldn't have because all these feelings are completely normal. As parents we put way too much pressure on ourselves anyway, this doesn't need to be compounded by rainbow baby guilt.

It's a strange place to find yourself when you have a rainbow baby. I didn't feel like part of the mummy crew because I struggled to relate to women who hadn't experienced any difficulties. I felt like women who hadn't gone through any sort of trials or setbacks didn't get it. I felt so secure in the pregnancy loss community because these women did get it, they did understand. Having said that, I could no longer be a part of the TTC and pregnancy loss sisterhood because even though I felt like I still belonged there, I didn't. It was not fair on those still waiting for their rainbows. The last thing they needed was me flaunting my new baby when they were so desperate to have one themselves. I know, I have been on the other side and even if you are told how tough someone had it and how long and arduous their journey was, you still don't want to hear about it because they have the one thing you are so desperate for. I soon found my feet in my new role as Mummy and I have focused on providing support and a story of hope for those in the midst of their journeys.

ABOUT YOU

What has been the hardest part of your journey so far?
Why? Answer this as honestly as you can. Write it as if
nobody else will ever read it. You may find that opening
up completely will help heal any deep wounds you may
have covered up, on the surface at least.

BACK TO REALITY

Spring was a complete blur of calmness and cuddles and then came summer. We were so busy, I felt like I was trying to make up for lost time and I wanted to create all the memories that I had imagined we would already have by now. I had spent years watching others make memories with their children and dreaming about being able to do it myself. Now was my chance. I didn't want to get to the end of maternity leave and regret that I hadn't made the most of it. As it turned out, day to day we didn't really do anything spectacular. We went to baby classes, ate more cake, met friends for more coffee and went on more doggy walks. Other than this, our daily outing was usually to the supermarket. I soon realised that it didn't matter what we did or where we went. All that mattered was that he was happy, safe and loved. Coming to this realisation helped to take the pressure off. I am a great believer in the saying 'happy mum, happy baby', after all it is difficult to be patient, kind and loving when you are tired, hungry, bored and stressed. I made sure I looked after myself and did what I needed to be able to be the best mum and wife I could be. At first, I would enjoy a few hours off every so often to do things like get my lashes done, have a pedicure or go to watch my netball team play. For my birthday in June I went out with friends for a curry. I was still breast feeding at the time so escaped after Bertie's evening feed. We had a couple of cocktails at a bar and then had a long dinner eating a mountain of Indian food and drinking giant bottles of beer. It was about 11pm by the time the meal was over. I walked in the front door, expressed some milk, gave Bertie a dream feed and was in bed before 12. Gone were the days of going 'out out' and that didn't bother me one little bit. I was so content with my little life and family.

I breastfed until about four months and was rather proud of this achievement. I know the advice is to do it for longer but honestly I was surprised that I was able to manage it at all. I really wanted to be able to breastfeed and was always going to give it a good go, but I have one nipple that has always been flat and the other has never been particularly perky. Pregnancy had made my boobs, and consequently my nipples, triple in size. In the recovery room after the caesarean I was assisted to latch Bertie on. I had been to a breastfeeding talk at the hospital, but I had no idea what to do and just let the midwife do what she needed to do. I tried it myself, but I struggled. My tiny new-born baby was rooting around trying to find something to latch on to, but my boobs were so swollen and the nipples so flat that it was like he was trying to latch on to a balloon. Back on the ward the midwife on the night shift helped too. My nipples were being tweaked, milked and even syringed by the staff, in order to get the all-important colostrum for Bertie. I continued to struggle with the latching on when we got home but persevered in between a couple of small pre-made formula bottles. It was actually with the help of one of my friends who has four breastfed children of her own that I was able to 'master it'. She came over to meet Bertie when he was five days old. I was emotional, had rock solid boobs and Bertie clearly wasn't getting what he needed from me. She walked in told me to get my boobs out and latch him on. She could see why I was struggling. I had some nipple shields in my collection of baby things that I had been gifted but I had never considered using them because I thought they were just there for if you had sore nipples. Mine weren't particularly sore and due to the nipple shape on the silicone shield I had assumed they wouldn't help me anyway because my nipples were so flat. I put them on and it was like magic. Bertie's suck literally drew my nipples out and the milk started flowing. It was quite reassuring to be able to see the magic white stuff in the shield. I will be forever thankful that my friend came to visit that day. Other than a short episode of mastitis, my breastfeeding journey was non-eventful and thankfully we were able to combination feed so had the best of both worlds. Scoop was also giving him a bottle of formula milk in the evenings to top up any deficit and this worked well for us because it gave them some bonding time and I was able to get a good block of about six hours sleep. I would go to bed after his evening feed at about 8pm and Scoop did the next one about 11/12pm and that would mean I wouldn't be required again until about 2 or 3am. We gradually introduced more bottles until July when he was just having a morning and evening feed from the boob. I had a brief moment of guilt when I first stopped breastfeeding but was able to stop myself from dwelling on it. I was conscious of putting pressure on myself and wanted to avoid indulging these feeling of inadequacy and inferiority after having dealt with them for so long.

We had Bertie christened at four months and it was a big celebration, by default really. The pub garden we chose to use for refreshments afterwards accidently double booked so there was a band on in the marquee next to the one we had reserved. It made for a good knees-up and it was so special having everyone there to celebrate with us. Over the course of the summer we got away as much as possible, to make the most of my time off. We visited family in the West Country, went on a fantastic camping trip to Dorset, attended Bertie's first festival CarFest and then had a trip to Spain to visit my dad in September. It was really special spending this time together and getting to know our ever-developing baby B. I also managed to wangle a couple of girly weekends away. I went to a hen do in Dorset and then to Center Parcs two weeks later with the girls. They were lovely breaks which allowed me some time to chill with good friends and focus on me. I think Scoop also really enjoyed having these weekends at home with Bertie, he was growing up so fast.

By the time the summer came to an end I started thinking about going back to work. I needed to speak to my boss and organise logistics. Oh how I loved maternity leave. I spent years watching colleagues go on their maternity leave, some of them multiple times so I wanted to make the most of mine. However, financially there would come a time when it was more sensible for me to go back so I did my sums and booked to go back at the beginning of January when Bertie would be 10 months old. We planned a trial of four days per week, to be reviewed after three months, taking into account my stress levels, our finances and the childcare situation. Originally, I had wanted to go back to work three days per week. I was one of those people with the opinion of 'why bother having children if you are going to get someone else to look after them all the time?' I take it back. It will be good for all of us, plus financially we are limited with our options. Also, the biggest lesson I have learnt in motherhood is to do what suits you and not to judge if others do it differently.

While I started thinking about my return to work from maternity leave, I began wondering if and when I would be able to do this again. *By 'this' I mean mat leave, baby, pregnancy.* Having a big family with lots of children has always been a dream of mine. Although I guess I hadn't really thought about actually trying for another baby because I hadn't been convinced that we would even manage to have one. Considering all that we had been through it was something that we needed to discuss with each other and really think about whether we could put ourselves through it all again. As soon as we started talking through our feelings it was clear that we were both fully on board. Not only that but we wanted to start trying as soon as was reasonably possible. We wanted a small age gap. When Bertie was six months old, I saw my specialist at Epsom Hospital. I took Bertie with me so they could meet him. After discussions with the team it was decided that I should have repeat blood tests done, in case the antibody was still present, but I would be prescribed the standard medications in the meantime. This was the same protocol that I was treated with previously and most importantly, successfully. It was left up to us to decide when we wanted to start trying for baby number two but was advised that we should ideally have at least a year between pregnancies so that my body would have time to recover.

I would really have liked to go back to work pregnant but that was not the case. Who knows how long it will take us to get pregnant and if that pregnancy will even stick. It is different this time though. The worst thing about recurrent pregnancy loss was not knowing if I would ever become a mum. Now that I am it is okay. I don't mind if it takes a bit of time to fall pregnant because I know that *it can happen.*

ABOUT YOU

We have no control over our age, medical history or genetics but there are some things we can control. Some things to consider:

- Nutrition
- Smoking
- Weight

- Caffeine
- Alcohol consumption
- Drug use

_____

_____

_____

_____

_____

_____

_____

_____

_____

_____

_____

Have you made any lifestyle changes to help with fertility? What sorts of things have you yet to try that might be helpful?

A LETTER TO MY SON

Monday 6th January 2020

To my dear little Albert

I write this letter to you on your first day of nursery. I am busy sorting some things out for my first day back at work tomorrow and the house is very quiet without you here, although your furry brother Cooper is keeping me company.

I just wanted to write you a little note to say thank you for a few things.
You made all my dreams come true when you made me a Mummy. You have been such a wonderful baby and so easy to look after. I have had the absolute best 10 months of my life being your Mummy. We've had lots of fun, made lots of friends and been to some lovely places.

It's a shame that I have to go back to work, but I think it will be good for both of us. You are going to love it at nursery and I think you will enjoy some time playing with friends and meeting new people. When we see each other now it will be extra special and I will give you lots of kisses and cuddles. I will look forward to bath time and reading you a story at bedtime and I'll be sure to plan some fun things for us to do on my days off.

You have been a real blessing in my life, more than you will ever know and I am so proud to call you my son. It's been wonderful to watch you grow and reach your first milestones. I was with you when you blew your first raspberry and when you rolled over, sat and stood for the first time. You have even started walking around with the little baby walker you got for Christmas and you can say mama and dada too! You are a clever little boy Albert, that is clear already. You are such a happy soul, so placid and funny and you have the absolute best smile and laugh. It melts my heart.

You are meant for great things Bertie and I for one am so excited to see you grow up (but not too fast though please).

All my love
Always

Your Mummy
XXX

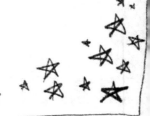

ABOUT YOU

Do you have a rainbow baby or an angel baby? Are you still trying for your baby or did you have one before this particular journey began? Write a letter to your baby; be they here with us, gone to soon, never made it to Earth or yet to be created.

MEN AND THEIR GRIEF

I am aware that I have written this book from my perspective and I know that it is important to consider the partner. I asked Scoop to write a chapter for the book but he's not very good at expressing himself, so we've had a chat instead. I've written something about how I think men can be supported when enduring miscarriage and recurrent pregnancy loss. I hope it is helpful.

I don't think that men usually get as broody as women do. However, I imagine that once a couple has made a decision to have a baby, the man will start to picture their life as a dad. They'll think about taking their little princess to the park and pushing her on the swings or teaching their 'mini me' to kick a ball for the first time. They'll imagine helping them with their homework, having lazy days together watching their favourite childhood films and simply being a happy family. That is the dream, right?

However, this end goal is not achieved so simply for some and the 'getting pregnant bit' can be as tough on men as it is on women. You assume that it will happen soon after you start trying but sometimes it doesn't. When it doesn't, your sex life soon becomes very regimented and you'll find that you are not allowed go to the pub with your mates because she is ovulating and has scheduled you in for some 'sexy time'. Not to mention the rollercoaster of emotions and feeling like you are constantly treading on eggshells through fear of triggering an upset or stress.

Like women, I think men also struggle to deal with feelings of guilt and embarrassment when they have difficulties conceiving. Is it my fault? Why is it not happening for us? Is there something wrong with me? Men can feel that their masculinity is in question if they cannot get their partner pregnant and this can result in negative feelings toward her and himself.

Then it happens. That positive pregnancy test. They may even be lucky enough to see the heartbeat on an ultrasound scan. Your imagination starts running wild and you develop real hopes and dreams for your future as a family.

And then it's gone.

The heartbeat is gone. The baby is gone. Your hopes and dreams for the future are gone.

You grieve.

As a couple you are devastated and inconsolable and as a woman you may also be dealing with the physical pain and hormonal emotions. But we often forget that men can also find pregnancy loss very difficult to deal with. A man is meant to be tough, handle their emotions, be strong, practical and support their partner. Men typically are fixers, but you cannot fix a miscarriage. They will feel hopeless, helpless and powerless as they observe the emotional and physical pain that their partner is going through and realise that there is nothing they can do to fix it. So instead they will go through the motions of taking care of their partner and focusing on all the other things which need to be dealt with such as household chores and liaising with family.

There is usually lots of support for women. They will have friends and family popping round, sending messages and bringing flowers. They'll cry and be cuddled by everyone around them. Men, on the other hand, will usually put a brave face on and act like they have everything under control but really they might also be struggling with grief. They'll often feel unimportant and invisible at this time.

Everyone has their own way of expressing their feelings and dealing with grief. Some men might not want to share how they are feeling with anyone other than their partner. They may throw themselves into something to try and forget (at least for a little while) what has happened. They may spend more time at the gym, doing DIY or go out for a drinking session with their mates to drown their sorrows. It's okay to grieve separately, it might be exactly what is needed. However, it is important to grieve together as a couple and have an open dialogue about how you feel. After all you are the only ones who truly understand the extent of your loss. Be kind and support each other in whatever way is right for you.

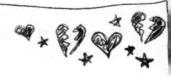

ABOUT YOU

Are you and your partner completely open with each other about how you feel? Or are you holding back to try and protect each others feelings? Have you considered writing these feelings down and showing each other. You wouldn't have to show each other if you didn't want to. Like I have previously mentioned, writing can help you to process and make sense of your emotions. It can be beneficial even if no one else ever sees it.

A letter to my partner _____

_____

_____

_____

_____

_____

_____

_____

_____

WORDS OF ADVICE FOR SUPPORTING THOSE WHO ARE NAVIGATING THIS JOURNEY

I know that it is incredibly difficult to know what to say or do for couples who are childless (not by choice) and particularly when they experience losses. I only really know what has helped us and I will share that with you. Before that though, it is probably worth suggesting what NOT to say in these circumstances. People often mean well but just don't know what to say. They end up blurting out inappropriate statements which are not intended to hurt but can be really insensitive. Here's what not to say.

Everything happens for a reason.

Sometimes shit things happen for no reason at all. If someone got cancer would you say this?

It was probably meant to be.

This is hurtful. Even if it was not a viable pregnancy, it is still heart breaking and it is not what they will need or want to hear right now. It provides absolutely no comfort at all, however true it may be in some cases.

At least you know you can get pregnant.

I heard this several times. The outcome is still the same. I am childless. Getting pregnant seven times has not resulted in having a baby, so how is getting pregnant any consolation at all?

It will all be fine next time.

You don't know that. Of course you hope it will, but you don't know. Also, what about this time? They wanted *this time* to work.

It'll happen when you stop trying so hard or you are thinking about it too much.

I've tried to 'stop trying' and it is near impossible. After tracking my cycles for so long I know them inside it out and can tell exactly when I am ovulating. How can someone just stop thinking about something that they so desperately want?

You're getting too stressed.

Recurrent pregnancy loss, and infertility for that matter, is incredibly stressful. It causes the stress; it's not a result of it. Blaming the losses on stress will make her feel like it is her fault and she may begin to blame herself. There is no evidence that shows that stress actually causes miscarriages.

You're still young; you've got plenty of time.

It doesn't make the losses any easier to deal with. I was 27 when we started trying for our family and I planned on having four children. I didn't have Bertie until the age of 33. As maternal age increases, so do the risks of miscarriages and other pregnancy complications. I doubt we will manage four even if we wanted to now.

At least it was early.

Don't try and put a positive spin on things, there is nothing positive about it. By minimising the loss you invalidate their grief.

It was just a ball of cells.

Is this meant to be a good thing? From the second you get a positive pregnancy test you have real hopes, real dreams and real plans for that baby. The grief is real!

I know that all these words are well meant and come from a good place. They are intended to bring comfort but unfortunately they often come across in the wrong way. That is usually due to awkwardness and not knowing what to say. Here are some helpful things to say. You could try these instead.

I am so sorry!

Simple yet effective.

I know how much you wanted that baby! I wish I could take your pain away and make things better for you.

Really there is nothing that anyone can do to make the situation better as no one can bring the baby back. By acknowledging the loss and heartbreak it shows that you understand that they are grieving and appreciate the extent of their loss. The loss of the pregnancy and the future hopes and dreams associated with it.

Do you want company?

Make contact, don't shy away. Take a bottle of wine round, take her out for a coffee or simply send a card. She might like the distraction of chatting about other things. However, do ask her how she is and how she is coping, she will open up about the loss when she is ready and if she wants to. It's good to talk and important to let the emotions out.

How can I help?

How you can help will depend on the sort of person they are, your relationship with them and on the circumstances of the loss. After the ectopic operation I really appreciated the lunches people brought round and the offers of dog walks while I recovered from the operation. Following other losses, I have just wanted to get blind drunk and cry at 3am in the kebab shop!

I'm here for you both.

Listen to her vent and remember that he will be hurting too. Message or call the following week to check in on them and let them know that you haven't forgotten about what happened. They won't ever forget and the grieving process can be long. It is comforting to know that you are not the only one who remembers.

The couple themselves will not be the only ones grieving. People close to them will also be suffering. The grandparents-to-be will have had their own hopes and dreams for the baby and the loss is theirs too. Close friends and family will also be finding it tough. They will be trying to provide support at this time but will feel helpless, wishing that there was something they could do to make everything better.

Everyone will react differently to pregnancy loss. You may worry about saying the wrong thing. If you do, I am sure they will understand that you didn't mean to offend. The worst thing you can do is ignore that it ever happened and say nothing at all! Just try to be there to support them and listen to how they feel. Acknowledge the loss, empathise and most importantly, be kind.

ABOUT YOU

Are you a member of any support groups in your area or on social media? Have a look and see if there are any that might suit you.

_____

_____

_____

_____

Are there any other books that you have read and would recommend to others navigating this journey? Or are there any that you might like to read?

_____

_____

_____

_____

_____

ACRONYMS

AF – Aunt Flo (period)

BD – Bed Down / Baby Dance (have sex)

BFP - Big Fat Positive (positive pregnancy test)

BFN – Big Fat Negative (negative pregnancy test)

CTG - Cardiotocography (foetal heart monitoring)

EPU – Early Pregnancy Unit

ERPC – Evacuation of Retained Products of Conception

HCG – Human Chorionic Gonadotrophin (pregnancy hormone in blood)

LMP – Last Menstrual Period

PAL – Pregnancy After Loss

PMP – Partial Molar Pregnancy

TTC – Trying To Conceive

TV – Trans-Vaginal (internal scan AKA light saber up the foofie)

TWW – Two Week Wait

SMM – Surgical Management of Miscarriage

REFERENCES

Lang, K., and Nuevo-Chiquero, A. (2012). 'Trends in Self-Reported Spontaneous Abortions: 1970–2000', *Demography*, 49 (3), pp. 989–1009.

NHS. 2018. *Diagnosis: Miscarriage.* (Online) Available at: https://www.nhs.uk/conditions/miscarriage/diagnosis/. (Accessed 16 September 2020).

Tommy's. 2018. *How common is miscarriage?* (Online) Available at: https://www.tommys.org/pregnancy-information/im-pregnant/early-pregnancy/how-common-miscarriage. (Accessed 16 September 2020).

Tommy's. 2018. *How long does it take to get pregnant?* (ONLINE) Available at: https://www.tommys.org/pregnancy-information/planning-pregnancy/how-get-pregnant/how-long-does-it-take-get-pregnant. (Accessed 16 September 2020).

Tommy's. 2019. *Tell me why.* (ONLINE) Available at: https://www.tommys.org/our-research/tell-me-why. (Accessed 16 September 2020).

Tommy's. 2020. *Early miscarriage and ectopic pregnancy may trigger post-traumatic stress disorder.* (Online) Available at: https://www.tommys.org/our-organisation/about-us/charity-news/early-miscarriage-and-ectopic-pregnancy . (Accessed 16 September 2020).

Tommy's. 2020. *Recurrent miscarriage.* (ONLINE) Available at: https://www.tommys.org/pregnancy-information/pregnancy-complications/baby-loss/miscarriage/recurrent-miscarriage. (Accessed 16 September 2020).

AVAILABLE SUPPORT

Miscarriage Association

The Miscarriage Association is here to provide support and information to anyone affected by miscarriage, ectopic pregnancy or molar pregnancy.
www.miscarriageassociation.org.uk
01924 200 799

Tommy's

Tommy's is the largest charity funding research into the prevention of baby loss. They support parents and families who lose a baby, experience premature birth and help everyone have a safe and healthy pregnancy.
www.tommys.org
0207 398 3479

Kicks Count

Kicks Count is the UK's leading baby movement resource and awareness campaign.
www.kickscount.org.uk
01483 600 828

Mind

Mind is a mental health charity that provides advice and support to empower those experiencing a mental health problem.
www.mind.org.uk
0208 519 2122

ABOUT THE AUTHOR

Laura Buckingham is a wife, mother, nurse and blogger. She has been on an incredible journey to start her family, dealing with recurrent miscarriage and pregnancy loss.

She started blogging to help process her thoughts and emotions during some of her darkest times but soon found that it was helping others too. Many people reached out to Laura and it was clear that her story could provide some hope for others who were on similar journeys.

She has also joined forces with another miscarriage mumma to create a podcast named 'The Worst Girl Gang Ever'. It focuses on open and honest conversations surrounding miscarriage and pregnancy loss.

Laura lives in Kent with Scoop, Bertie, Cooper the dog and Ernie the tortoise.

She hopes this book will help you navigate your own journey and that you enjoy reading her memoir.